Family Systems Application to Social Work: Training and Clinical Practice

Family Systems Application to Social Work: Training and Clinical Practice has also been published as *Journal of Independent Social Work*, Volume 5, Numbers 3/4 1991.

The Haworth Press, Inc., 10 Alice Street, Binghamton, NY 13904-1580
EUROSPAN/Haworth, 3 Henrietta Street, London WC2E 8LU England
ASTAM/Haworth, 162-168 Parramatta Road, Stanmore, Sydney, N.S.W. 2048 Australia

Library of Congress Cataloging-in-Publication Data

Family systems application to social work : training and clinical practice / Karen Gail Lewis, editor.
  p. cm.
  "Has also been published as Journal of independent social work, volume 5, numbers 3/4, 1991" — T.p. verso.
  ISBN 1-56024-191-8 (H : acid-free paper). — ISBN 1-56024-194-2 (S : acid-free paper)
  1. Family psychotherapy. 2. Family social work. I. Lewis, Karen Gail.
RC488.5.F3337   1991
616.89'156 — dc20
                                                              91-26307
                                                              CIP

Family Systems Application to Social Work: Training and Clinical Practice

Karen Gail Lewis
Editor

The Haworth Press, Inc.
New York • London • Sydney

Family Systems Application to Social Work: Training and Clinical Practice

Family Systems Application to Social Work: Training and Clinical Practice

CONTENTS

ABOUT THE EDITOR

Karen Gail Lewis, EdD, ACSW, who has been practicing family therapy for over 20 years, is currently in private practice in Washington, D.C., and on the faculty of Johns Hopkins Medical School, Child and Adolescent Psychiatry. She has taught family therapy to mental health professionals in graduate schools, community mental health agencies, hospitals, and public and private schools. The co-editor of *Siblings in Therapy, Life Span and Clinical Issues* and editor of *Variations on Teaching and Supervising Group Therapy,* Dr. Lewis is currently working on a textbook on the overlap between social work, family therapy, and the urban poor. She has published numerous articles and book chapters on family therapy, gender issues, and the urban poor, and has presented papers both nationally and internationally. Dr. Lewis is on the editorial board of several professional journals, and is book review editor for the *Journal of Independent Social Work.* She has a masters degree in social work, a doctoral in counseling psychology and school consultation, and is certified as a clinician and supervisor of marriage and family therapy and as a group therapist.

Family Systems Application to Social Work: Training and Clinical Practice

Introduction

Karen Gail Lewis

Social work is unique among the other mental health disciplines with its dual emphasis of policy and clinical practice. Social work's origins are in social action, with the early friendly visitors, and later settlement house workers who were concerned about reforming conditions under which the impoverished and emotionally and physically handicapped people lived.

With the advent of Freudian theory, social work moved to establish credibility among the other mental health professions and began helping people understand their internal conflicts and better adjust to their life situations. Social work had moved from social reform to personal adaptation. The war on poverty renewed the focus on social action, but the split in the field remains, the battle between generic and specialization. Are we a clinical or social justice profession?

> . . . Should social workers continue to devote as much effort as they do to ameliorating the human consequences of undesirable social and economic conditions? Would it not be preferable for the profession to devote all its energies to changing the conditions that seem to create these problems at least as rapidly as social workers can ameliorate them? (Briar, 1977, p. 1531)

I believe, as do the contributors to this issue, that the duality of purpose is what makes social work so powerful. However, the potential of the integration of these two components has not been maximized. Students learn the theory of policy and social justice but the clinical courses are based in individually oriented psychotherapy. Social work has theory for understanding the context of the lives of poor, underorganized, ghetto, often minority families but, unfortunately, no specific clinical theory for working with them. Social workers in the field lack professionally rele-

Karen Gail Lewis, ACSW, EdD, is in private practice and on the faculty of Johns Hopkins School of Medicine, Department of Child and Adolescent Psychiatry, 1107 Spring Street, Silver Spring, MD 20910.

1

vant tools to impact in any significant way on people with emotional problems or to help them understand how their real life problems create the emotional ones. If therapists do not recognize when people's behavior is a means of adapting to their life situation, they may interprete the behavior as pathological.

> The more popular psychotherapy treatment theories, with their emphases on pathology, are non-systemic and use a diagnostic base that is irrelevant, ineffective and insulting to poor people, particularly people of color. They overlook cultural differences and values and seek to find causes of poor people's problems in their intra-psyche. Extreme poverty and homelessness can affect people's feelings about themselves, make some "crazy" and leave many more feeling helpless, powerless, and despairing. (Parnel and VanderKloot, page 7 of this issue)

> The underorganization of these families grows more out of their social context than any pathology specific to individual families. Underorganized communities spawn underorganized families. (Aponte, p. 25 of this issue)

SOCIAL WORK AND FAMILY THERAPY

For some inexplicable reason, there has been an antipathy between family systems (family therapy) and social work.[1] Family therapy is a way of viewing rather than a technique for dealing with a situation or interaction. Family therapy has added a more systemic understanding of individual and family roles and patterns connecting over the generations. Family systems concepts fit well within the person in the environment framework, adding the extended family and the social community. The adversarial relationship has been a loss to both disciplines. Structural family therapy has its origin in working with the same population of disenfranchised people as do social workers; several other schools have techniques that are immensely helpful for working with families living in chaos. Is it coincidence that (a) the National Association of Social Work was established in the 1950s, the same time family therapy was beginning; (b) one of the pioneers of family therapy was a social worker, Virginia Satir; and (c) among the organization of trainers of family therapy (American Family Therapy Association), more than half have a masters in social

---

[1]This may be more true in the schools of social work than in the field.

work? Despite the apparent antipathy between the two fields, I am pleased to note that there seems to be a move among female family therapists to return to their roots, owning their social work origins. This is in large part, I suspect, influenced by the developing influence of the feminist movement.

These Families

"These families" and "this population" are families overwhelmed by a social environment that provides little emotional, social, and economic support. They have euphemistically been called many names: low-income, poor, inner city, multi-problem, dysfunctional, disorganized, minority. By labeling these families, we dehumanize them. However, there needs to be a way to talk about this specific population of people so that we can acknowledge and address their unique situation. So, for the sake of clarity (and until a more accurate term is established and widely recognized), all of these labels are used interchangeably in this issue; no bias is intended.

From the social worker's perspective, these families require a tremendous amount of physical and emotional investment with few rewards. They overwhelm social workers with their multitude of problems; they often appear to lack effort and interest in bettering their lives. They are families that perpetuate for generations a series of social problems such as teen pregnancy, drugs, crime, unemployment, welfare. The abundant services provided seems to have little effect. After a length of time working with this population, burn out is high, as is disillusionment and cynicism.

From the family's perspective, they are beleagued with poverty, crime, disease, lack of education, unemployment, and few resources that, if available, could substantially help change their lives. They live with the stigma of racism and classism, with no expectation that things can really be different. They often lack a dream of a different reality for themselves. They see social workers as intruders, invaders of their world. While they may have an occasional caring one, their general view is that social workers cause more harm than good; they accuse them of being bad; they blame them for their situation. They come from the outside and offer suggestions with no real appreciation for what it is like to live inside the ghetto.

Within the family therapy world, the term isomorphism means a pattern that repeats itself on different hierarchal levels. Social workers' frustration, hopelessness, and cynicism isomorphically are experienced by the recipients of social services. Clients are angry and frustrated in dealing with governmental agencies, hopeless in ever bettering their lives, and

cynical that social workers really care. You may be caring, but the last
five . . .?

THE NEED FOR SOMETHING DIFFERENT

The articles included here should raise the poignant question of how we
as professionals can help those who live in a very different world, where
daily survival is a chore. How can we distinguish between what is pathological and what is adaptive when people live in a community that is often
likened to a "war zone"? What is needed is a broader picture, a new
paradigm for working with this population — a paradigm that encompasses
the worker, the client, the extended family, the community, the government — a paradigm that understands the context in which people live and
sees behaviors as attempts to adapt to impossible situations. Social work
and family therapy together provide a perfect marriage for creating an
ecosystemic theory and practice model.

> A focus which draws boundaries too narrowly around individuals or
> families leads to treatment goals which primarily involve accommo-
> dation; an ecosystemic approach necessarily leads to the analysis of
> larger systems including political systems as an integral part of treat-
> ment. (Walker & Small, page 80 of this issue)

What does all this have to do with the social worker in independent
practice? Can't we escape from having to deal with these issues? Simplis-
tically, "If you aren't part of the solution you are part of the problem."
More specifically, we are the teachers, the supervisors, the role models,
the leaders. We need to understand and teach; we need to see the connections between the "inner city" and the larger society. What happens in the
isolated poor inner cities today forebodes the tomorrows of the suburbs.
Systemically, we can not live in isolation, keeping our heads in the sand
and hoping if we don't see it, it won't touch us. The fall out effect of
disintegrating urban communities will eventually spill over and touch everyone. We can not hide our heads and assume it is not our problem.
Further, we have a social obligation to see what is happening and if not
speak out publicly, speak up within our smaller professional world. That
is part of the social work ethic.

OVERVIEW OF THIS SPECIAL ISSUE

The articles here are not intended as a comprehensive overview of working with inner city, underorganized, culturally diverse people. Hopefully, they will act as a scanner, showing a range of social situations that social workers confront. The topics chosen are not all inclusive, but they do represent many of the more common situations. The first section of the book is focused on teaching and training at all levels: social workers with undergraduate degree, graduate degree, post graduate training. The first article, "Family Systems Thinking and the Social Work Dean," sets the stage for thinking about the larger systemic context in which we live and work. Ray Bardill speaks as a dean of social work, looking at family/systemic concepts that are important across the various hierarchies in the work family.

Tonti, in "Teaching Family Systems Therapy to Social Work Students," presents a model for teaching family systems in a graduate school of social work. As often happens, her course on family therapy is an elective, a separate course from the on-going clinical practice course. She uses a parallel (or isomorphic) model of learning, showing how students face the same issues families do as they struggle with the one-down position, ambivalently seeking new ideas.

Aponte, in "Training on the Person of the Therapist for Work with the Poor and Minorities," describes his training model for professionals who already have their graduate degree. This would include master level social workers who want to learn family therapy, specifically as it relates to working with multi-cultural poor, underorganized families. He presents a framework for his training and shows how he has students face their own biases and personal issues in working with this population.

The last article in this section, "Training Social Workers in Public Welfare: Some Useful Family Concepts" by Flashman, presents a training model for teaching family therapy concepts to welfare workers and case managers. She emphasizes four concepts most relevant to their work with employment: family context, single parent mother, use of positives, and rituals to mark change.

The second section covers specific clinical situations frequently encountered by social workers. The first article, "AIDS, Crack, Poverty, and Race in the African-American Community: The Need for an Ecosystemic Approach" by Walker and Small, presents an incredibly painful yet clear image of one segment of our population. They then present a treatment model for this community, emphasizing the necessity of having it community based and led, where residents are a part of the identification of the need for and creation of their own programs.

Tracy and McDonell, in "Home Based Work with Families: The Environmental Context of Family Intervention," describe a modern day version of the friendly visitor. Home based workers are trained to assess and intervene from an eco-systemic perspective. In addition to the extended family focus, the physical and social environment are considered crucial in the assessment and treatment.

In "Doing with Very Little: Treatment of Homeless Substance Abusers," Berg and Hopwood describe using Solution-Focused Brief Therapy in their study of substance-using homeless adults. They inquired what type treatment and services the homeless wanted and needed. The authors do not offer happy ending stories, but they conclude with specific suggestions for treatment.

Another hidden group of social work recipients are the mentally retarded. "The Community Residence as a Family: In the Name of the Father," by Fenby, describes one unrecognized result of the transition from hospitals to living in the community: the administration represents power and repressiveness, and inadvertently perpetuates residents' childlike and dependent roles.

Lewis presents a model for helping families re-unify after foster care placement. "A Three Step Plan for African-American Families Involved with Foster Care: Sibling Therapy, Mothers' Group Therapy, Family Therapy" is an approach aimed at countering the high rate of recidivism. Before seeing the family together, the siblings work on identifying their role in making the reunification work and the birth mothers learn and practice executive skills.

Hartman, in "Every Clinical Social Worker is in Post-Adoption Practice," addresses a frequently unacknowledged topic — adoption. Social work participates in the silence around adoption by not recognizing that adoption touches birth parents, adoptive parents, adoptees and all their relatives. She discusses the two major themes — loss and identity — and discusses implications for practice.

Another painful and often hidden issue in practice is wife abuse. In "Shame and Violence: Considerations in Couples' Treatment," Balcom, uses a shame-based theoretical framework, discusses the interaction of shame and violence, describes the different types of shame cycles, and shows how shame effects the male development. Four stages of treatment are presented.

The last article, "Mental Health Services — 2001: Serving a New America," by Parnell and VanderKloot, presents a clear picture of life in the inner city—for the social worker and the clients. Using family systems and Chaos Theory, the authors present an empowerment-based treatment model for the urban poor, and combining both components of social work. They conclude with a social and political challenge to social workers in independent practice.

Many of the articles are disturbing; they may make you angry or anxious. We believe that is good. Social work is not a complacent field; it grew out of a need for social justice and reform; unfortunately, today's society still has these same needs.

TRAINING

Family Systems Thinking
and the Social Work Dean

D. Ray Bardill

With the emergence of systems thinking in the late 1950's as a theoretical base for working with family problems, new perspectives and new methodologies for treating dysfunctional family situations emerged. For social workers, family group interviewing provided one way to operationalize the "new systemically" oriented treatment approach (see Bardill and Ryan, 1969; Bell, 1961; Satir, 1967). The presence of an entire family unit in the treatment interview opened opportunities for a wide range of treatment strategies and techniques. In the ensuing years, expansions in theoretical considerations provided additional approaches to the emerging practice of family therapy (see Haley, 1976; Minuchin, 1981; Satir, 1972). For instance, the use of the two-way mirror and phone in supervision are treatment strategies which have added to the range of systemically based treatment possibilities. As the depth and breath of systemic thinking has evolved, its usefulness has expanded well beyond the realm of family therapy. Systemic thinking has permeated much of the theoretical basis for the profession of social work. Social work's person-in-environment

D. Ray Bardill, PhD, is Dean, School of Social Work, Florida State University, Tallahasee, FL 32306. He is also President, American Association for Marriage and Family Therapy, Washington, DC.

perspective has been greatly enhanced by systemic thinking (see Germain and Gitterman, 1980).

Since 1979 I have used systemic thinking to refine my knowledge, understanding and skills in the art and science of both family therapy *and* academic administration at the level of dean of a school of social work. The reciprocal learning that has taken place from the wide range of experiences in both spheres has been beneficial to me both as clinician and as a dean. While the context for a family therapist and the context for a dean are clearly two distinct professional domains they both contain similar systemic dynamics.

A school of social work has all of the systemic characteristics of a social context. Like a family, a school of social work is an aggregate of people with all the active dynamics of any set of human systems. While a school of social work is not kinship based, it carries an ever evolving life history complete with stories to justify that history. Faculty members serve as historians for consciously, and unconsciously, promoting the continuation of the existing systemic rules for a particular school of social work. A school of social work has various overlapping systemic triangles such as dean/faculty/students and higher administrator/dean/faculty. As a system, a school of social work shows organizational tendencies, specific boundary characteristics and has its own unique communications style.

The purpose of this article is to consider how parts of systemic thinking may be used by a dean to establish a specific work-place atmosphere for a school of social work. While a dean may attempt to create a specific work-place atmosphere, the nature of any work environment is the result of the interactions between and among the people and structures involved; hence, any atmosphere is co-created. The particular systemic perspective used for this discussion will be referred to as the relational systems model. This version of systemic thinking is based on my interruption and expansion on some of the fundamental ideas of Virginia Satir (1967-1972) and John E. Bell (1961). As its basic theme the relational systems model posits that:

1. Human beings exist in a complex web of influencing relationships with each other and with multiple overlapping social contexts.
2. All that exists may be accounted for within the (a) human realities of (reality = what is) self—the personal dimension, other—the interpersonal dimension and context—the social systems dimension and (b) the spiritual reality—the life connection to the creator of the universe.
3. All realities contain the possibilities for enriching the positive

growth and wholeness potential of human beings as well as their context.

4. The primary job of all helpers (therapists, teachers administrators, etc.) is to assist people to identify the growth and wholeness possibilities that exist for them in all of their realities.

THE SOCIAL WORK DEAN

"One of the toughest jobs in university administration" is a colleague's description of a school of social work dean's job. In the book *On Minding The Store: Research on the Social Work Deanship* (Gandy et al, 1977) written over a decade ago, the authors state "during the past few years deans of graduate school of social work have left their posts at a rate which in the eyes of some observers, has been alarming." Although the rapid turnover for social work deans seems to have abated somewhat in the recent past, the job continues to be one of the most difficult and challenging in academic administration.

About deans in general, Tucker and Bryan (1987) say, "all these roles that academic deans must, at various times, assume in fulfilling the leadership responsibilities entrusted to them by their institutions and respective colleges, schools or divisions" (Preface 1). They go on to say, "Viewed from afar by aspirants, the dean's job may appear to be glamorous and easy but our microscope will reveal more than glory and happy times (Preface 2, 1987). After reviewing his seven years as a dean, Harry Sultz (1989) says, "I can better appreciate the words of Warren Bennis and Burt Nanus in *Leaders: Strategies for Taking Charge*. 'It's not easy, you know, learning how to lead. Its sort of like learning how to play the violin in public. Unfortunately the discordant notes seems to linger long after the melody has faded.'"

In addition to the expected responsibilities of all academic deans such as budget management, personnel decisions, student academic advising, curriculum concerns, wider university relationships and fund raising, the social work dean most often heads a nondepartmentalized professional school or college. The implications of such an arrangement are that, for all practical purposes, the dean assumes the tasks of both dean and department chair. Thus, the social work dean is embedded in, and has critical responsibilities for, two powerful and demanding systemic levels. As a result social work deans, like department chairs, are largely in direct daily work contact with faculty, staff and students. In addition to these "front line" responsibilities the social work dean must carry out the university wide responsibilities expected of all deans. Deans interact with the various units of the central university administration. Positive links with key people in central administration are vital to the ongoing success of a professional school. In the overall scheme of things social work, in comparison to medicine, law, business, engineering, etc., is not likely to enjoy a high status within the university hierarchy. This means that considerable time and effort will be spent establishing a positive position for the school of social work within the larger university system.

As an academic representative of the profession of social work, local, state and national commitments become part of the dean's expected responsibilities. Experience has shown that effective social work deans must be active in a variety of groups in order to gain and maintain the respect of professional peers. And by virtue of their position, deans often are expected to assume leadership positions in various associations and groups.

Effectively managing the varying time demands becomes an integral part of a social work deans job. In a recent national survey of social work deans, Munson (1988) found that deans work an average of 54 hours per week in their administrative position. In my opinion the average number of work hours worked per week is well beyond 54.

FACULTY RELATIONSHIPS

Negotiations between and among the various sub-systems which make up a school of social work are often difficult and time consuming. Social work faculty members themselves, including the dean, reflect the diverse nature of social work interests. It is not unusual for a social work faculty to be split on just what the mission and objectives should be for their school. The dean must somehow provide clear direction for the school while taking into account varying faculty interests, goals and commitments.

Both the Munson (1988) survey and the 1977 findings of the Gandy, Randolph and Raymond study (Gandy et al. p.39) identify faculty relationship issues as a major contributing factor to the difficulty, unpleasantness, and stress of the position of a social work dean. In reporting the most unpleasant tasks performed, 64% of the deans listed a task specifically relating to faculty (Munson 1988). In the monograph *Counsel for New Deans: Observations on the Deanship*, (Leon W. Chestang, 1988) twenty-five social work deans were asked to give advice to newly appointed deans. Almost all of the deans identified and gave some advice about the complex human relationships dimension of a Deanship. Clearly, the quality of human relationships is a major factor in the nature of the work-place atmosphere of a school of social work.

It might be noted that the overall importance of the dean-faculty relationship in creating a functional work-place atmosphere is not limited to schools of social work. Sultz, (1989) in the earlier mentioned article, lists aspects of the dean-faculty and faculty-faulty relationships in all but one of his principles; (1) deans cannot change the academic behavior of faculty members, (2) deans cannot personally effect significant institutional changes based on priorities or values different from those prevailing among the faculty members (3) deans cannot be the driving force behind major academic achievement, (4) deans can be effective only as a facilitator, or enabler for others, not as the orchestrator of programs and (5) deans can productively put energy into creating a positive image for the school/college and program. "Academic image is often more influential than the reality of an institution" (Sultz, 1989). Gandy (Gandy et al., 1977) points out that in many situations facts are of little consequence, the way it seems is all that counts. In the final analysis effective deans give attention to the relationship factor as a major consideration in the work-place atmosphere in an academic environment.

SYSTEMIC CONSIDERATIONS

It is my contention that a relational systems approach may provide the basis for specific guidelines to be used in setting up a specific work-place atmosphere in a school of social work. Very simply, the relational systems model is based on multi-systems view of family dynamics. Like a family, a school of social work is multi-systemic in nature. Specifically, the personal, interpersonal and contextual dynamics each in their own way exert its own powerful influences on the larger systemic whole – the school of social work. As such, certain systemically oriented principles provide guides for the conduct of both family units and academic units. Each principle is congruent with the basic propositions of the relational systems model presented earlier. The five principles are: (1) structure and roles are for the purposes of organization, not control (2) humans experience lineally and explain cybernetically (3) a systemic understanding of the strong relationships between leadership and roles is critical to effective administration (4) systemic thinking involves attention to the personal, interpersonal and total unit dynamics (5) the organizing concept for all of the above relational systems model principles is found in the systemic notion of worthness. While each of the above principles stands on its own taken together they provide the basis for a particular approach to academic administrator, or therapy.

First Principle – Following is a guiding principle about organizations and structure that has been of enormous help to me over the years. The principle is *structure and roles are for the purposes of organization, not control.* As such, organization and structure provide for the integrity of the system and facilitates the carrying out of the tasks necessary for a school to accomplish its stated mission. Individual roles provide an organized set of expectations for the people who occupy specific labeled positions. Knowing who is to do what when and where serves to empower the faculty, administration and the school. For instance, it would be chaotic for everyone involved as well as the school as an organization if specific roles and role expectations had to be negotiated every Monday morning. Clearly, the integrity of any social system requires some stability of roles and organization.

Much like a family therapist, a systemically oriented dean is sensitive to the use of structure and roles as a basis for power plays by people within the school. However, in functional systems, the outcome of organizational processes will reflect "what-fits" for both the people involved *and* the mission of the school. Power maneuvers emanating either out of structure roles or personal motives require immediate attention of the dean (Chestang 1988, p. 39).

At the interpersonal, or horizontal level, faculty members' relationships to each other form patterned sequences which are influenced by personal, interpersonal and context considerations. The vertical relationship dynamics are furnished by administrative roles, faculty ranks, staff designations, student statuses and organizational characteristics.

Second Principle — A second guiding principle simply recognizes that *humans experience lineally and explain cybernetically.* Thus, my immediate thought response to an event is that *A* caused me to do behavior *B*. For instance, when a recent graduate has contributed $1,000 to our foundation fund following a phone call from me, my immediate experience was "my phone call did it!" Yet, to fully explain why he/she contributed the money requires a more extensive examination of such activities as years of fund raising, phone calls, and changing techniques for informing our graduates about the need for foundation money and the graduate's particular life situation. A dean who considers only the linear part of the ongoing dynamics of a school will be stuck in the stimulus — response considerations of a highly complex human system. It takes just a bit of imagination to think of the results of administrative decisions based in strict cause-effect thinking. The complexity of a School of Social Work demands systemic thinking.

Third Principle — It is necessary for a dean to have a systemic understanding of *the strong relationship between leadership and roles in the creation of an effective work-place atmosphere.* The overall leadership of the system is provided by the dean, associate dean or an assistant dean. Like all systems, leadership is required, and questioned. Like family roles, academic roles are defined by the surrounding context. All roles carry a defined set of expectations, responsibilities and functions. Labeled roles affect what a person thinks of himself/herself and what other people think of him/her. Much like the therapist role, the dean is responsible for the *overall* conduct of the system. The view-from-the-top of the dean is based on a total system perspective. No one else in the academic unit is charged with the overall responsibility for the school. Like family members, faculty, staff, and student roles are more specifically defined. Expected actions for everyone are generated out of structure, labeled roles and accompanying expectations.

As with family dynamics, role confusion leads to system dysfunction. Faculty members or deans who are unable to maintain role integrity are like children who assume a parental role or parents who assume a child's role. Family therapy has long included the restructuring of family role relationships as a major therapeutic strategy. Experience suggests that role confusion often is a source of system problems for both families and academic units; or, to put it another way, a wheel that tries to act like a motor will likely disable the whole car.

One consultant, after visiting a particular graduate school of social work, commented to the dean, "You have 20 assistant deans don't you?" Clearly, the faculty has its role and administration has its role. While close cooperation and support between and among all roles is essential, the blurring of roles carries a high probability of system dysfunction. Likewise, deans who attempt to maintain a faculty role will likely get into structural difficulties very quickly. Such deans are thought to be interfering with curriculum decisions or practicing cronyism with certain faculty members.

Certain actions are generated out of the expected role of dean. Generally, deans are responsible to central administration for budget, personnel and specific academic type decisions relating to students. Some of the administrative decisions are painful to specific faculty, staff, or students. Excellence in academic administration demands that difficult decisions be made with sensitivity toward the people involved. However, like therapists, deans are required to make decisions that give appropriate priority considerations to the overall purpose of the context. Humans are not perfect and as such, mistakes are made by everyone. When a person is confronted by a dean about specific actions, the person has a choice about how to use the confrontation. Some people use confrontation to grow and improve while others regress and become more problematic. Experience confirms over and over again that while leadership is important at all times, it is vitally critical when things are not going well. The true importance of leadership shows when difficult tasks, confrontations and decisions are required.

In each of their respective roles deans, faculty and staff decisions are required which may be aversive to a particular person. For a dean, part of his/her role is to promote and maintain high morale but it is not the role of a dean to keep everyone happy (Chestang 1988). Faculty members have a similar responsibility especially in the area of advising and grades. Difficult leadership decisions are, simply put, difficult decisions. Handling difficult decisions well in all roles is desirable but does not eliminate the essential negative nature of some decisions.

Like the leadership of the therapist, academic leadership is a combination of art and science. To use a paraphrase from Tucker and Bryan (1987, p. 3) a dean, (and *all* other faculty, staff and students) is a leader who uses science in the performance of an art, an art that finally defies precise analysis. Like therapy leadership, academic leadership serves best when it allows for an environment which enables everyone involved to choose to grow, create and realize their full potential. In other words, a goal of leadership is to empower everyone in a particular area of responsibility. In evolving a positive work-place atmosphere the effectiveness of leadership is a fundamental factor. At all system levels it is the leadership quality that directly impacts on the vision, purposes and ability to turn a desired stated goal or dream into a reality and to do so with the active cooperation of others in the system. However, like in family therapy, leadership qualities in a school or college always co-evolve within the particular academic unit. Or, in the others words, *overall* leadership is provided by the deans *and* leadership directed to *specific* responsibilities and functions is provided by faculty, staff and students. An abdication of the defined leadership responsibilities by any part of a system will contribute to system wide dysfunction. In this respect, the role of the dean carries with it co-responsibility for insuring that leadership is present in the various parts of the work-place setting.

Fourth Principle — Appropriate systemic thinking requires *simultaneous attention to the personal and interpersonal dimensions as well as total unit dynamics*. This principle is especially directed to the dean who in his/her enthusiasm for seeing the whole fails to notice the individual people and the way these individual people interact with each other. In this article *appropriate* means that all of the dimensions of total reality have been given the attention required by the uniqueness of the situation the specific people involved and their relationships with each other.

For some reason, personal considerations are sometimes given inadequate consideration in a systemic perspective. Each member of a school of social work is a unique human being. While personal characteristics may be given descriptive terms such as caring, mature, open, aggressive, mean, friendly, immature, loner, etc., there is an elusive intangible quality about the personal dimension. At the same time humans exhibit amazing consistency in their behavior patterns. Even people who are inconsistent are habitually inconsistent, or to put it another way each person brings himself/herself into every situation. The systemic context for a school of social work will bring out each person's unique way of dealing with others in organizational settings. Effective deans know about and understand the uniqueness of each faculty member. Faculty members are amazingly predictable in their way of responding to issues and situations.

Equally important are the interpersonal patterns of the various dyadic and triadic relationships between and among faculty. The hierarchial arrangement, and the accompanying labeled roles, inevitably carry the baggage of unresolved, or the freedom of resolved, family/authority issues. Faculty members, staff and deans alike act out their respective functional or dysfunction life scenarios in the human interplay of deceit, honesty, rebellion, responsibility, arbitrariness and openness, etc. In systemic thinking the power of interpersonal dynamics applies to all hierarchial levels, roles, and persons. In other words, it is as important for each faculty member, staff person, and student to provide effective interpersonal leadership in his/her *specific* area of responsibility as it is for deans to provide excellence in *overall* interpersonal leadership area.

For better or for worse, the interpersonal part is an active ingredient in the actions, influences and responses generated by all members of a school of social work. All of the generally accepted characteristics of emotional maturity such as accurate self-awareness, empathy, openness to different perspectives, actions that reflect congruency with a sense of purpose, non-judgmental, integrity in the domain of responsibility, attraction to the positive, etc., or the lack of any or all of the above, play themselves out in the interpersonal dimension of a school of social work.

Deans, or therapists, who fail to model honesty, empathy, caring, and understanding in their relationships are likely to experience difficulty at the personal and interpersonal levels. Those deans who assist others to turn problems into possibilities will find they do not have to deal with as many problems. Satir was once reported to have noted that if the therapist developes possibilities, the problems will go away.

Fifth Principle—The organizing concept for all the principles previously mentioned is found in a systemic view of worthness. Systemically, worth is a wholistic concept based in a recognition of the simultaneous worth of *all* human beings and the world around us. A worth position, or *worthness, attends to the value of the personal, interpersonal and context levels of the system as a whole*. Thus, a goal of worthness is to discover and energize the dimension of positive value of all system levels.

Attention to the worthness dynamic in the academic setting is reflected in subtle, yet conscious, efforts to recognize and acknowledge the positive motivations, contributions and actions of everyone in the school of social work. Life experiences confirm the fact that every event experienced by human beings is evaluated for its impact on worth. The recognition of the power of worth is exemplified in *The One Minute Manager* in the suggestion to "catch people doing something right" (Blanchard, p. 19). To put it another way, people are most productive when they sense positive value in what they and their colleagues do and in what their organization is contributing to our world. Systemically, this means that the tradition (systemic rules and institutional memories) of the work-place becomes one of active acknowledgement and recognition of the contributions made toward the various goals of the school.

Attention to worthness does not mean that mistakes, errors, or misdirections are ignored. It means that mistakes are confronted in a timely manner, specifically and with empathetic sensitivity. It is important to remember that the goal of negative feedback or corrective action, is to assist people to do their best in making a contribution to the school. Or, to put it another way, negative feedback is something you provide *for* someone and the school or college not something you do *to* someone. Virginia Satir, over and over again, recognized the importance of the positive frame for all interactions, even negative feedback. Clearly, the time when humans need love and understanding is often the time when they deserve it the least.

Systemic feedback also means that the dean is open to the same quality of caring negative feedback from a faculty member. Administrators who insulate themselves from corrective communication will not enjoy the benefits of negative feedback; mistakes will go uncorrected.

For everyone, a sense of value comes from making positive contributions to the goals of the organization. Constant attention to the worthness factor is required and serves as an organizing concept for a positive workplace atmosphere.

LEVELS OF CHANGE

At this point in my understanding of systems dynamics, several ideas seem fundamental to me. First, accounting for total-unit dynamics is a primary responsibility of the dean. No one else is in a position to take the overall view of the entire academic unit. Identifying and relating to systemic dynamics allows a dean access to critical forces at play at systems level. Second, while change at system level is necessary it never comes easy; change is painful. Deans, like family therapists, are part of the change process and as such must absorb some of the pain of change. Third, system-wise deans openly recognize the requirement for change in an academic unit. However, like the family therapist, the *dean's* vision of change is general rather than specific. The specifics of change for a school, like a family, evolve from within the total unit not from the dean. The contribution the dean makes is to provide the academic environment and general direction which helps people think for themselves. Neither effective social work deans, or family therapists, operate through a power perspective which takes away the opportunity for others to learn about what they are doing and to grow from it.

Deans can be helpful in creating the context for changing "institutional memories." Actively reframing past events as well as allowing "new histories" to emerge can provide the impetus for ongoing change within the system. For instance, a dean can be instrumental in providing a series of opportunities for people to disagree without negative consequences. He/she can use modeling behavior to establish an ethos of intentional empowerment for faculty and students.

Experience, as a dean, and a family therapist, leads me to offer words of caution about change to *any* dean. In the beginning stages of a deanship it is vitally important to distinguish between a true honeymoon period with the faculty/students and a true crisis situation. A true crisis situation allows the opportunity for substantial systemic change. Crisis theory has taught us that people react to a crisis with an openness to new possibilities. A dean, like a family therapist, may be able to use the crisis situation to encourage major needed changes in the overall academic program. At the same time, how often have we heard the lament of a recently dismissed dean who thought he/she had been brought to a school by a higher administration in a time of crisis to "change things." Extreme caution is needed in such situations. For one thing, the crisis may not be located in the school of social work. The location of the crisis may be in the system level called higher administration; in such situations the dynamics of crisis do not apply to the school of social work.

Even a honeymoon period between a new dean and his/her faculty is *not* likely to be powerful enough to allow for dramatic programmatic changes. It is like an exaggerated positive beginning relationship with a family therapist. It must be handled with care. The positive relationship/honeymoon will end abruptly if the change process moves too quickly.

On the positive side, a new dean may come into the school excited about the prospects for positive change in the school. Recruitment interviews with higher administration and faculty likely were filled with words pointing to challenges for a future. Openness to change seemed so real. However, like families who seek help with a problem, change *is* wanted *and* feared. System-wise deans understand and use the positive momentum of the honeymoon period to make whatever changes the system will tolerate but the major effort is put into setting up the process and structure for change *in the future*. Critical to this change process is to project notions about a plan and a strategy for change. However, the idea is to talk about change without being specific. Like the family therapist, the dean is required to know the difference between a crisis situation, a mislocated crisis situation and an exaggerated positive relationship/honeymoon period.

Giving attention to the personal, interpersonal and total unit dynamics requires that a dean project the notion that he/she will be around for at least 4 to 5 years. Like a family system, an academic system relates best to the idea that leadership will be around for the near future. The building of a relationship between the dean, higher administration and the faculty takes time, effort and a sense of permanency for the whole system. Simply put, everyone involved reacts to a known "short-timer" in a different manner than they do to a permanent dean. The importance of relationship building diminishes when it is clear that the dean will not be around long.

Finally, there is a universal quality to the interpersonal dynamic of gratitude that, if recognized, may avoid some strong negative feelings between deans and faculty/staff. It is critical to know that in general there is a wide gulf between the experience of personal gratitude *toward* another and the personal expectations of gratitude *from* another. Deans who expect gratitude, or thanks, for the helping hand given a faculty member/staff likely will be disappointed. Simply put, humans are not likely to feel gratitude for help received for very long. Clearly, all of us have been helped by key people in our professional progress and most of us regard the help as "deserved." Yet, how many times have deans complained about the ingratitude of faculty and staff. Family therapists and deans alike are able to understand that "whatever you do for your kids, your spouse, your subordinates, your boss, or your friends (your clients) just remember: you'll be a lot happier if you think of it as doing it for yourself. And then try like hell to forget you did it because the beneficiary has" (MacKay, 1988). Clearly the demand for a sense of personal worth leads most of us to regard ourselves as primarily self-made people. The sense of dependency which often accompanies a feeling of gratitude is discomforting to most people. System-wise deans understand the interpersonal implications of the dynamic of gratitude and follow MacKay's advice.

SUMMARY

Relational systems thinking provides the basis for a wide range of notions about dealing with many of the administrative problems faced by social work deans. With some variations the same systemic elements are operative in both the academic work place and the family therapy situation. The basic multi-systems dynamics relating to the personal, interpersonal, and context are the same for both domains. When these multi-level dynamics are examined from the systemic perspective a number of guiding principles for a deanship emerge. It is my contention that when a social work dean thinks, feels, and acts in terms of a worthness driven multi-systems perspective the probabilities for an effective and empowered School of Social Work are greatly increased.

REFERENCES

Bardill, D. R., Ryan, F. J. (1969). *Family group casework*. Washington, D. C.: Catholic University of America Press.

Bell, J. E. (1961). *Family group therapy*. Washington, D.C.: Public Health Monograph, No. 64, U.S. Public Health Service, Department of Health, Education and Welfare.

Chestang, Leon W. (1988). *Counsel for new deans: Observations on the deanship*. Miami, Florida: Prepared for a workshop sponsored by the National Association of Deans and Directors of Schools of Social Work.

Gandy, John T., Randolph, Jerry L., and Raymond, Frank B. (1979). *On minding the store: Research on the social work deanship*. Charleston, S.C.: College of Social Work, University of South Carolina.

Germain, Carel and Gitterman, Alex. (1980). *The life model of social work practice*. New York: Columbia University Press.

Haley, J. (1976). *Changing families*. New York: Gardner Press, Inc.

MacKay, Harvey. (1988). *Swim with the sharks*. New York: Ivy Books, p. 239-240.

Minuchin, Salvador. (1981). *Families and family therapy*. Cambridge, MA: Harvard Press.

Munson, Carlton. (1988). *Dean/director survey summary of results*. Fordham University, N. Y.: An unpublished survey report.

Satir, Virginia. (1967). *Conjoint family therapy*. Palo Alto: Science and Behavior Books.

Satir, Virginia. (1972). *People Making*. Palo Alto: Science and Behavior Books.

Sultz, Harry A. (1989). "Had I a chance to be a dean again, here's what my principles would be." *Chronicle of Higher Education*, May 31.

Tucker, Allen and Bryan, Robert A. (1987). *The academic dean: Dove, dragon and diplomat*. Tallahassee, Florida: Unpublished.

Training on the Person of the Therapist for Work with the Poor and Minorities

Harry J. Aponte

America's poverty is not the destitution of widespread famine and starvation of the third world. It is a poverty in which the basic structural underpinnings of society are collapsing, leaving its citizens with overwhelming emotional stress and few social supports. Today, this societal illness permeates all strata of society with the greatest weight pressing on the poorest.

Families are breaking up. More children are born outside of marriage. Women are raising children alone. Violence of all kinds is increasing. Drug abuse is an epidemic. Communities are disintegrating. This is today's America, a society which both poor and minority clients and their therapists share.

With today's violence and abuse in families growing, for example, the problems clients bring to social service agencies and mental health clinics are getting uglier. These problems are more acute among the poor. The stark reality is that the ills socially disadvantaged families present to therapists today appear more daunting than ever.

Social service workers and therapists are supposed to help. They train to work with family dysfunction and emotional illness. They even receive training with their own personal issues that impede their work. However, where the need is most acute, for their work with the poor, therapists get relatively little help. There are relatively few therapeutic models that address social ills together with emotional problems. There are few societal and agency supports for the individual therapist's efforts. There is little help for the therapist trying to cope with the emotional stress and personal demands of work with poor, underorganized families so many of whom are also minorities.

Harry J. Aponte, ACSW, is Director of the Family Therapy Training Program of Philadelphia, Academy House, #32D, 1420 Locust Street, Philadelphia, PA 19102.

We need to think not only about medicines for America's strain of poverty, but also about preparing the healing to administer those medicines. This paper, will touch on a therapy that is ecological in nature. It will offer a professional training model that recognizes the special needs of therapists working with underorganized families, especially among the poor and minorities.

THE ECO-STRUCTURAL APPROACH

When we work with low-income families, the obstacles to good results are many. Minuchin (Minuchin, Montalvo, Guerney, Jr., Rosman, Schumer, 1967) developed the structural approach to family therapy out of a need for a therapy suited to the poor, especially the hard core poor. Because troubled communities are a source of these families' troubles, the eco-structural approach (Aponte, 1979) broadened the model to include the social ecology of the community. It incorporated the community with the family in the expanded model's theoretical and technical frameworks (Aponte, 1976b).

Family Underorganization

This article is not about well-functioning poor families. It is not about the economically indigent, who otherwise have a sound family and community life. It is about poor families who cannot manage their family relationships and life tasks. It is about families crushed by the effects of poverty—*underorganized families* (Aponte, 1976a).

Social and economic deprivation and pressures have undermined the basic structure of the underorganized family. These are fragmented families that have incomplete hierarchies, with partially articulated roles, and emotionally truncated relationships. The family does not have an adequately evolved system of values to hold it together and guide its relationships and actions. Consequently, the family loses the sense of its own identity and power. It is like an individual with a deficient immune system, vulnerable to infections from its environment. The poor, underorganized family is susceptible to the social evils of its community. The organism breaks down and, in turn, becomes a carrier of the infection. These families suffer terribly, and pass on their troubles to their children and back to their communities. They not only become victims, but also potential victimizers.

When these families come in for help, whether voluntarily or involuntarily, the lack of family organization is often the most immediate reality a therapist faces. More often than not, these families have one parent at home, usually a woman. The absent father's involvement is inconsistent, if it exists at all. Roles in the family are often ambiguous, with the mother not a consistently effective executive and administrator in the family system. She lacks the ability to define and enforce a systematic family organization. She has trouble directing her children. The family is groping through its life tasks. Everything feels difficult.

These families are trying, struggling, having some successes, but too many failures. It is not that they have no rules, that is, no organization. Their efforts to survive translate into some kind of family organization. However, their family structure lacks the definition, elaboration and/or flexibility to cope with the demands of life. These families present not so much a *dis*-organized family as an *under*-organized family.

The Family's Community

The underorganization of these families grows more out of their social context than any pathology specific to individual families. Underorganized communities spawn underorganized families. The larger society starves local neighborhoods of social and economic supports. Eviscerated, the community cannot generate a vital social structure with the social values that give life to its communal soul. In turn, the community cannot nurture its citizen families. Families who survive these communities, often do so not because of, but in spite of, their communities.

Many of our clients' neighborhoods are economically depressed—with poor housing, high crime, failing schools, few jobs and inadequate governmental resources. There is often a shortage of effective leadership from within the local population and from their politicians. The community may compromise its values—for example, accepting a drug trading economy as inevitable. It is not that these neighborhoods do not have any resources, but that they are few and hard to access (Aponte, 1989).

America's legacy of racism stifles and crushes many of these poor, underorganized communities consisting of racial and ethnic minorities. Race is so much a part of American culture that it defines and organizes personal, societal and economic relationships. Inevitably, racial biases, hatreds and tensions become internalized in people's views of themselves and society.

However, even where American public policy is supportive of the universal rights of racial and ethnic groups, it, paradoxically, discourages cultural difference. Public schools, for instance, present a homogenized culture. They do not reflect neighborhood values and culture for fear of excluding anyone. Our society has not solved the problem of guaranteeing the right of individuals to equality while protecting the need of communities to claim their own social structure. Community life has been sacrificed for universal rights, national economics and national culture.

As a result, what suffers in these neighborhoods and families is their system of values, the ethos that knits people together. A cohesive value system in a community fosters the structural integrity of families and hope in the individual. That common belief system sustains life through good and bad times.

However, the vitality of this ecology of values among a community, its families and individual citizens is as delicate and complex as any ecosystem. Everyone has a part to play in forging those values, including mental health and social service institutions. Psychotherapists, for example, are today's healers of the emotional life of families, and like schools, are shapers of the community's values. The professional community, with its own world views, competes with cultural values of families. For example, the social politics of family therapists imbue their work with families, offering models of family relationships that may or may not harmonize with the traditions of some ethnic groups. The helping professions support or undermine the infrastructure of values in communities and families.

A commitment to the poor must support the community-family ecosystem with the integrity of family life, and the cultural and economic vitality of their communities. Ideally, any therapeutic approach to low income families will claim an ecological perspective.

An Eco-Structural Solution

Therapy for the chronically poor must deal with,

1. the immediacy and concreteness of their problems,
2. the structural organization of the family,
3. the values of the family and its community,
4. the community resources of the family,
5. the links between family and community.

One therapeutic model that attempts to meet all of these requirements is the *eco-structural* approach.

Technically, the eco-structural model attempts to work with all family members and community institutions that are part of the problem and potentially part of the solution. Eco-structural therapists view their clients as part of their community, and, when indicated, will set up meetings with all parties involved. For example, in a school related problem (Aponte, 1976b), a social worker may meet with a family and personnel from the school — the principal, teacher and counselor. The social worker looks for and works through a specific behavior or event that embodies the problems in the relationships among the child, parents and school.

In the eco-structural model, the therapist asks those involved to address the issue with one another in concrete terms in the therapist's presence (structural family therapy's *enactment* [Minuchin, Fishman, 1981]). The therapist looks to see how they relate around the problem. This gives the therapist a chance to study how the family organizes itself to solve problems. The therapist intervenes actively in the interactions among family members and community. The therapist works for a change, in his or her presence, aiming to achieve results right then that are palpable to the family and others. For example, in a family-school interview, by the end of the session, a worker would want them to be at a different position than when they started, at the very least, agreeing on a new problem solving strategy.

When a family is severely underorganized and in crisis, it may also be necessary to start therapy with an extraordinarily intensive effort. Many of the home based models of therapy have adopted an approach that calls for concentrated work over a relatively short period of time, usually between four and eight weeks (Kaplan, 1976). In the eco-structural model, this intensive effort with a complex and, possibly, underorganized ecosystem of family and community, demands a team of at least two therapists.

Moreover, the therapeutic team requires active institutional backing from its agency or clinic. Ideally, the agency will integrate organically with the structure of the community. It will find ways of operating from within the community that will mobilize resources for their therapists' work with their client families. It will seek out an already existing, or help organize, a forum where community and local government representatives can meet to plan and talk. The governing body of the agency, together with the director, would be active in this network. The agency's commitment to the community begins at the highest level.

In the neighborhood, the agency can also organize multi-family groups from families receiving service from the agency. They can be sources of daily support for the member families. These multi-family groups become part of the network through which therapists do their work.

The eco-structural approach attempts to bring together families and community, with therapists and their agencies. This is an effort at an ecological solution to an ecological problem. Integral to this approach is that, conceptually, the ecological network (the therapeutic system) includes the therapist.

THE PERSON OF THE THERAPIST

All therapists contend with their personal selves in the therapeutic process. They bring their emotional, familial and social issues into their work. Along with personal family history, their social class, economic status, ethnicity and race also affect the attitudes and behavior of therapists. Moreover, on top of their own personal agenda, therapists wrestle with their reactions to their clients' behavior, all of which Freud called *countertransference* (Freud, 1964).

Classical psychoanalysis called for a detached and passive stance in therapy, with therapists keeping their feelings private. This minimizes analyst interaction with a patient. In contrast, today's active therapists involve themselves more personally with families; their responses are less private. The therapist has less insulation from the dynamics of therapist-patient interactions. The constructionist perspective goes even further. Lynn Hoffman (1990) says, "A second-order view would mean that therapists include themselves as part of what must change; they do not stand outside" (p. 5). Working with low-income families, by its very nature, calls for a greater than average active involvement because therapists have to supply more of themselves to the entire therapeutic effort.

The underorganization in many poor families calls upon therapists to offer more help with communications and with organizing functional family structures. The urgency and concreteness of families' personal and social problems also require therapists to involve themselves actively in pursuing solutions. The community itself will entangle therapists in negotiating between families and institutional bureaucracies. From any and every perspective, therapy with the poor is an active affair for therapists.

Underlying this entire process of therapist involvement in clients' lives is the therapeutic relationship and its personal components. Like anyone else, therapists and clients have to negotiate distance, control, and content in their relationship. The poor, in general, and poor minorities in particular, present therapists with common human relationship issues, as well as special social and cultural issues, which can greatly complicate the therapeutic relationship. Wide gulfs may exist between therapists and the poor deriving from differences in economic status, race, education, life experience, life style, values, etc. This distance between them impedes mutual understanding, communication, and affective connections, i.e., the ability to collaborate in therapy.

These gulfs between therapists and poor families directly affect therapists' ability to diagnose, intervene and relate. Successful therapy will depend in part upon closing the gap enough to work with personal and social differences.

The Goals of Person Training

Therapists enter the therapeutic relationship with their own family life experiences and socioeconomic backgrounds, and all the troubles and successes that come with these histories. In order to pay "careful attention to the human element . . . [in] the essential relationship between the therapist and the family," says Nancy Boyd-Franklin (1990, p. 95), "we must first explore ourselves as people, as men and women, and [then] as therapists." Being anchored about their personal lives will be particularly important for therapists when working with families whose personal boundaries can be so diffuse and confusing. Being resolved about their socio-political issues will make it easier for therapists to contend with the powerful social issues intrinsic to their efforts with the poor and their communities. Speaking to the need for therapists to look at their own social context, Pinderhughes says:

> It is not possible to assist clients to examine issues concerning cultural identity and self esteem if helpers have not done this work for themselves. (Pinderhughes, p. 19)

From the base of their own family and social history, therapists will examine their clients' lives. They will look for common family and social experiences, along with what is new and alien to them. They will strive to develop their ability to identify with their clients. They will discover what they need to learn about their clients' life styles and culture. They will explore what they have not resolved for themselves about socially and politically laden issues in their clients' lives. Finally, they will understand how their own life experiences affect how they relate to their clients. From a sensitivity and from insight into themselves, therapists will build the capacity to relate to their clients and their problems.

Person Training for Therapy with the Poor and Minorities

Speaking of what therapists need in working with cultural differences, Pinderhughes argues that, "effective service delivery requires practitioners to develop cultural sensitivity that is characterized by flexibility, openness, warmth, and empathy" (p. 19). She advocates training therapists to resolve their issues around ethnic difference. However, working with poverty also adds class and income level to the challenges that confront therapists' cultural biases.

Having "good" attitudes about race and socioeconomic status is not enough. Who is to say what is the correct outlook? Training should not be cultural brainwashing. For work with socioeconomic and ethnic difference, therapists will need to develop clarity, security and conviction about their own personal and cultural heritage, as well as understand others. This will permit therapists to be more empathic and open to others, as well as critical and strong, to share power, as well as hold their own. The ultimate purpose of person training with a societal facet is to help therapists use their personal life experience and socio-political perspectives to do better therapy with the poor and minorities.

The therapy, itself, particularly with the socially disadvantaged, brings together in the therapeutic process personal psychology, family dynamics, and social reality. Person training of therapists serving the poor should mirror this complex of perspectives. Therapists aim to achieve greater conscious mastery of their own personal and social dynamics in the therapeutic process as they relate to and work with disadvantaged families.

Integrating Personal and Clinical Training

If training on the person of the therapist is to develop a practitioner-therapist, then it should run in conjunction with clinical training. To this end I will describe a person training model applied through the eco-structural therapeutic model which are both tailored for work with the poor. In a training for work with low-income families, a *personal-social-clinical* (PSC) approach incorporates the ecosystemic realities of a family's life into the therapist's clinical framework.

Two training approaches exemplify the components of a personal/social-plus-clinical training experience. They are Elaine Pinderhughes' "experiential group model" (Pinderhughes, 1989) and the Aponte/Winter "person-practice model" (Aponte, Winter, 1987).

Pinderhughes pursues personal understanding in the therapist, "by exploring within a group format the participants' own feelings, perceptions, and experiences vis-a-vis ethnicity, race, and power" (p. 211). The model emphasizes the "in vivo" experience in the group. It deals not only with attitudes, but also with interaction across cultural difference. It looks at values "on both personal and societal levels" (p. 212). This sharing in the group context around the interpersonal dynamics within the group is extended through *discussion* to practitioners' clinical work (p. 240).

The Aponte/Winter person-practice model complements Pinderhughes' approach. In common with the "experiential group model," the base setting for training the therapist is the trainee group. The person-practice program works with therapists' life issues, including their values, but does not have Pinderhughes' exclusive and intensive focus on ethnic differences. Its emphasis is on therapists' personal family issues, and places a high premium on the practical clinical formation of trainees. Aponte/Winter person-practice training includes supervising the clinical application of therapists' personal work. The model uses live supervision as the ultimate, integrative experience.

The PSC training model accepts the same premise in person training for treating the poor, i.e., that it should be founded on developing clinical skills. Fundamentally, therapy with the poor must be practical and grounded in real, clinical experience. Therapists must be actually working with low-income families all during training. Clinical practice will give their training real life reference points, and provide them with a practical arena to test their learning.

Personal-Social-Clinical Training
Training Model

Presented here is an outline for a PSC training program based on the Aponte/Winter model and elements of Pinderhughes' model.

Composition of group:

- Number: 10 participants with terminal degrees in mental health or counseling.
- Mix: Ideally include trainees from the racial, cultural and socioeconomic backgrounds that reflect the make-up of the trainees' clientele.

Frequency and length:

- Two year program (first year stressing their personal issues of the trainees, including their family and ethnic backgrounds, and second year, stressing their clinical practice).
- Two day sessions convene monthly for 10 months (creating an intensive group experience with trainees during the two days).
- 7 work hours per day, with trainees eating meals and socializing jointly.
- Each two day session begins and ends with a 2 hour group rap.
- *Individual* 1 hour long presentations for each trainee to discuss personal or clinical issues through talk along or with audio/videotape;

leaders work directly with the trainee for 45 minutes, and then guide group discussion for 15 minutes.
- Live supervised 2 hour long *clinical* sessions, including a 1 hour interview and another hour split for discussion before and after the session.
- For both years, trainee makes 4 individual one hour presentations and receives live supervision or has a live consultation for 3 two hour sessions.

Leadership:

- 2 leaders (co-leaders).
- Ideally, the leaders are male and female; they have ethnic and socio-economic backgrounds reflective of the trainees and their clientele, or have experience with families that correspond to their trainees and their clients' histories.

Setting:

- Training center to be outside trainees' settings, protecting trainees' privacy.
- Commitment to confidentiality by all participants.
- Training center to have video and observation rooms.
- Training center to have agreements with trainees' agencies to supervise trainees live with their clients, and to have contact with the communities of the families.

Training Content

Trainees work on personal issues and clinical material both years, accenting the personal in the first and the clinical in the second. Within the framework of clinical practice, they work on their family history, personal and social values and relationship to society.

Family History

Trainees aim to identify personal relationship patterns and family issues that characterize their lives and, potentially, their work. They look at the issues they have had to overcome in their lives; where they succeeded and where they failed. They examine these family issues through presentations of their genograms and discussion of cases which give rise to their issues. They may arrange for one time only consultations with their own family members conducted by the trainers. (Trainees request these consultations when they want help exploring some issue with their families). They also look for their personal issues in the live supervision of their clinical interviews.

Value Training

Therapists may or may not be settled about the history of the evolution of their values. Trainees review the history of their personal and social values in their families and communities, for example, around religion or race. They put special emphasis on current struggles around their values. As part of their work, trainees may not only discuss value issues with family, but also with peers, such as in ethnic organizations, and social institutions, like churches. They will certainly look to identify value issues in their clinical presentations.

Training about Society

In training to work with the poor and minorities, therapists will examine their own and their family's social history. They will identify major themes in their relationship with today's society that may affect their clinical practice. Just as trainees may return to their family about personal issues, they may want to return to family to work out questions of heritage, race, gender and family socioeconomic history. Trainees may visit old neighborhoods, regions or countries of their origins. They may want to meet and talk with ethnic, racial or gender defined groups already organized for political, historical or personal support purposes. Looking at their clinical work from a social perspective will be essential to case presentations and supervision.

All these explorations about family life, values and society provide precedents and experiences which will serve therapists well in their work with the client groups they are to serve. Therapists will have personal maps to guide their inquiries into the family and social contexts of their clients.

Trainees' personal-social exploration will also serve as a pilot to their efforts to help clients look at social issues in the problems they present for therapy. Trainees will have a social perspective when trying to understand clinical issues. They will be sensitive to where and what interventions they need to make in a family's community — whether around welfare, jobs, housing, justice system, etc. Not only will "clinical strategies . . .

bring this wider [social] context into the consulting room" (Goldner, 1985 p. 23), but clinical interventions will take therapists out into the community.

The Formation of Personal-Social-Clinical Trainers

Of paramount importance are the leaders who will guide these trainees through the labyrinths of their personal and social histories. Just as therapists need to know where they are in their personal lives when helping clients with theirs, person trainers need to have done some serious work about themselves. Considering the triple level complexity that a personal, social and clinical experience will present, it helps for trainers to have had some life experience and clinical seasoning of their own. Personal therapy also deepens self knowledge and mastery. Training as a clinical supervisor broadens the trainers' therapeutic perspective. Finally, experience with low income and minority families in the community is essential.

Potential trainers would also do well to have gone through some form of person training, and to have apprenticed as trainers with experienced people. Leading training on the person of the therapist calls for considerable expertise as a therapist and clinician. It also requires possessing a method of pulling all those clinical, supervisory and therapeutic skills together to direct the clinical training of the person of the therapist.

One more word about a very basic challenge for the leaders of person training, especially when the training deals specifically with social issues. Therapists who gravitate toward social issues also are inclined to have strong political convictions. They tend to stand aggressively behind their beliefs. They often are activists, which can carry over into their teaching. Professional ethics restrain our pushing personal and social values on our clients, but they do little to protect trainees from our personal crusades. Regarding the influence of leaders in person training programs, I believe that trainees deserve the same safeguards clients have. There is no easy solution to the issue because the debate is heating up about how "to make the links between social issues and clinical practice even more explicit" (DeMuth, 1990). The question of how and when to introduce the social values of trainers into training should be considered as seriously in training as therapist values in treatment.

The Group

Lastly, one must highlight the use of group process in this training. The group serves several important functions. The most obvious is that by participating in the presentations of other therapists, trainees have the opportunity to learn from the experiences of others. Another, is that the group is a social context in its own right with all the caring, support, insights, perspectives, prejudices and divisiveness of any social group. The group offers a mix of people's psychology, life experience, ethnicity and socioeconomic backgrounds. Within the training program, the group creates another opportunity for trainees to learn about themselves in relationships and to improve themselves with the help of others. Trainees can address personal and social issues in the clinical relationships within the group.

The Story of a Trainee

Len is a social worker, a young African American with considerable professional skills and personal presence. He was one of two black trainees in the training group, the other was a woman. Because of his obvious personal attractiveness and air of competence, he commands respect and draws people to him. He is consistently friendly and gracious but acknowledges that he hides much inside, emotionally distancing himself from people.

Len did three particularly important presentations in his first year of the program. In the first he presented his genogram, and with it his life story. In his second presentation, he conducted a clinical session with his colleagues role—playing family members. In the third, he conducted a live session with a family.

Len is the third of six children. He described his mother as "warm, nurturing [and] accepting." His father was a tough man who "demonstrated [his strength] by [his] ability to experience hardship without a display of emotions." However, his father confused him because he was "fond of having philosophical talks with [him] about education, money and life in general." Len's conflict and shame were over the fact that during his childhood his parents had become emotionally estranged. His mother became an alcoholic and his father a philanderer. Len had grown up feeling protective of his mother and angry with his father.

Len took on the burden of the "responsible" son. He became the "hope" of his family, the one who would achieve. He was sent for a better education to military school. He was to be mostly among whites. As he told his story, there emerged the tension between his loyalty to his roots and his wish to fulfill his family's aspirations in the outside world. There was the boy who hid his pain and embarrassment about his family's problems from his own neighbors at home. This same boy had to cover up his self doubts and fears in that outside, often white, society which expected much of him. All this led to a man who avoided intimacy in relationships because he feared exposing his needs and vulnerability. He knew this was affecting his relationships with women and guessed it was impairing his therapy, although he was not clear how. Through the exploration of his genogram he committed himself in the training to do something about his "vulnerability as it relate[d] to [his] role as therapist."

The genogram work served to set the theme for his training. There followed two clinically oriented presentations that helped him get further into the work. The first was a role play in which he played therapist and several trainees played the family members. The trainers used the experience to interrupt the process at several points in order to ask the "family" members to feed back to Len how they were experiencing him. It was apparent Len was feeling pressured to perform and was becoming uptight in his fear of failing. His colleagues in the simulated family were able to tell him how unconnected they felt to him, how cool and rational he had become. These were his friends talking. It was a powerful and disturbing confrontation for Len.

In having to perform with the simulated family before the training group, he was dealing at some level with his family of origin, and at another with that outside world of school that was testing him. He had to be tough and competent in both. The discussion in the group about how he had changed with them, how they cared about him, and how accepting they felt about his very human struggles as a therapist gave him much needed feedback. He could talk it out with them, check out how they felt about him and ask for their emotional support. Len also chose to enter personal therapy outside the training group, a common decision made by trainees in the program.

In the next clinical presentation, Len brought in a family for supervision. He saw the family live with the leaders and group behind an observation mirror. Len brought in a white family with which he had been working. He felt he had a good relationship with this family, but knew he needed to push hard on some issues that would be threatening to the mother in this single parent family. He needed to help her stop being overprotective of her troubled and immature son. However, when confronted by Len in the session, she became defensive. Len just as quickly reacted defensively. Again he was being tested before his peers.

The training leader called him out of the session and got him talking about what was behind the woman's behavior, her fear of his criticism and rejection. The trainer helped him talk about his fear of failure and embarrassment. The trainer eventually had to join the family and Len in the session. He helped them talk about the trust in their relationship and the good work they had done together. They relaxed. The trainer left. Len was feeling safer and was able to pick up and help the mother to feel safer with him. In the face of her being a woman and white and of his having to be successful with her and before his colleagues, Len could still engage with her without the previous uptightness. Len was beginning to change his outlook and behavior in the context of his therapy.

In his second year, Len continued with his work on his family of origin. He had needed to get beyond his shame about his parents and, thereby, of his roots. He presented several times on his parents. That led him to look at both the good in his parents and their very human vulnerabilities, which they shared with the rest of the world, not just his family. His mother had been an exceptionally loving person, loved and appreciated by those who knew her in spite of the drinking problem of later years. His father had been a rock, supportive of his family and also the spur to his professional aspirations. His mother had died years before, but his father was still living. Len was coached to talk with him over a series of visits. To his amazement, once his father sensed safety in his son's genuine interest in talking with him, he showed himself anxious for a relationship with his son. Father opened up his own fears and vulnerabilities to Len. He released Len from the old image of the hard-face. Together, they also talked about Len's mother, understanding her in greater depth. Len translated his new personal family experiences into new experiences for the families he treated — white and black — and into his relationships with his clients, male and female. Len entered a doctoral program on graduating from the training program.

CONCLUSION

The poor and minorities of our communities come to us for service. Along with all the common problems of life, they also present personal and clinical issues that are special to their circumstances. They need help that is specially tailored to their needs, and the therapists and workers who serve them need training that specially prepares them for the job. This article focuses on a model for training the person of the therapist who works with low income and minority families.

Because a person training program will need to have a clinical focus, the eco-structural therapeutic model was offered as an example of a clinical framework for the training. In my opinion, any model of therapy or service that purports to serve the poor and minorities needs to have an ecosystemic perspective. The eco-structural model of therapy specifically serves the underorganized, poor family within a community context. It aims at solving concrete problems, reconstructing family relationships, and remedying social ills that directly impinge on client families. The model expects agencies to tie into the social structure of the communities they serve. It looks for therapists to work directly and actively with families and their communities. The model's perspective treats family and community as parts of an ecosystem that can generate and solve problems. It is an ecological therapy with psychological, familial, and social dimensions. It offers a broad framework for discussing person training for work with the poor.

The active involvement of therapists with the personal and social problems of poor, underorganized families demands a great deal, both clinically and personally, from therapists. Relating to these families and treating their special problems challenge therapists at the levels of their social values, and personal, ethnic, and socioeconomic backgrounds. Therapists' own personal societal experiences help or impede their work with these families whose race, culture and economic circumstances are often central to their personal problems.

To work with poor and minority families, therapists need a clinical training tailored to the problems these families face. They also require a training experience that prepares them personally to deal with the social issues working with these families will raise. The personal-social-clinical training model offered here uses co-leaders and a peer group experience in a two year program. It includes presentations by therapists about their personal life and clinical experiences. It culminates in supervision of their clinical work. The training aims to integrate the worker's person with the worker's therapy. The community orientation of the training helps therapists place their work with families in their clients' social reality, providing a truly ecological framework.

The personal-social-clinical model offers an ecological perspective to training the person of the therapist in working with poor and minority families.

REFERENCES

Aponte, H. J., (1976a). Underorganization in the poor family. In P. J. Guerin (Ed.), *Family therapy: Theory and practice* (pp. 432-448). New York: Gardner Press.

Aponte, H. J., (1976b). The family-school interview. An eco-structural approach. *Family Process*. 15:303-311.

Aponte, H. J., (1979). Family therapy and the community. In M. S. Gibbs, J. R. Lachenmeyer, & J. Sigal (Eds.), *Community psychology: Theoretical and empirical approaches* (pp. 311-333). New York: Gardner Press.

Aponte, H. J., (1985). The negotiation of values in therapy. *Family Process*. 24:323-338.

Aponte, H. J., (1989). Please join me in a short walk through the south Bronx. *AFTA Newsletter*, pp. 36-40, no. 37, Winter.

Aponte, H. J., & Winter, J. E., (1987). The person and practice of the therapist: Treatment and training. *Journal of Psychotherapy & the Family*. 3:85-111, Spring.

Boyd-Franklin, J., (1989). *Black families in therapy: A multisystems approach*. New York. The Guilford Press.

DeMuth, D. H. (1990). The social consciousness of family therapy: A time of change. *AFTA Newsletter*. 40:10-13, Summer.

Freud, S. (1964). Analysis terminable and interminable. In J. Strachey (Ed. and Trans.) *The standard edition of the complete psychological works of Sigmund Freud* (Vol. XXIII, pp. 216-253). London:Hogarth Press. (Original work published 1937.)

Goldner, V. (1985). Warning: Family therapy may be hazardous to your health. *Networker*. 9:18-23, Nov.-Dec.

Hoffman, L., (1990). Constructing realities: An art of lenses. *Family Process*. 29:1-12.

Kaplan, L. (Ed.) (1986). *Working with multiproblem families*. Lexington, Massachusetts: Lexington Books.

Minuchin, S., Montalvo, B., Guerney, Jr., B., Rosman, B., & Schumer, F. (1967). *Families of the slums*. Basic Books: New York.

Minuchin, S. & Fishman, H. C. (1981). *Family therapy techniques*. Cambridge, Massachusetts: Harvard University Press.

Pinderhughes, E. (1989). *Understanding race, ethnicity, & power: The key to efficacy in clinical practice*. New York: The Free Press.

Teaching Family Systems Therapy to Social Work Students

Roberta Tonti

This paper presents a format for teaching an elective family therapy course to graduate social work students. We will observe how systemic thinking within the class facilitates both the teaching and the learning processes. I will describe the process of teaching family systems in a way that reflects the same process as students working systemically with a family in treatment. As the students learn a new way to think about people and problems, we will see how this is reflected, in parallel issues, in their own experiences and in the experiences of their client families.

THE WORLD OF THE SOCIAL WORK STUDENT

A group of social work students has come together, in the grander scheme, to accomplish a goal—to earn a masters degree in Social Work. They come from all walks of life: they cut across a variety of socio-economic and ethnic groups; their ages span three decades; they have a range of clinical experiences; they bring varying expectations for their classes. At the end of their training they will have a masters degree, usually a large debt to repay, two years of field work, and a shaken sense of their knowledge base and expertise. Their expectation, as well as that of their peers and employers, is they are now the "trained professionals" who are sup-

Roberta Tonti, ACSW, LISW, is in private practice and also teaches part time at the Mandell School of Applied Social Sciences—Case Western Reserve University, Cleveland, OH. She is currently President of the Ohio Division of the American Association of Marriage & Family Therapy. Coorespondence may be addressed to: Roberta Tonti, MSW, 2120 South Green Road, South Euclid, OH 44121.

The author would like to acknowledge all of the students at MSASS whose participation and willingnwss to learn gave me the information and perspective to put this paper together.

41

posed to know what they are doing. They have shared, with their peers, the ups and downs of graduate school life, the various expectations, accomplishments and aggravations of school and field placement. They also share the task of having to rebuild a sense of their competence and expertise which has been challenged by two years of new information and experiences. They leave school feeling full of excitement, yet unsure of their new skills and their ability to maneuver in the professional world.

PATHWAY TO CHANGE
FOR STUDENTS AND TREATMENT FAMILIES

Teaching masters level social work students systemic family therapy is a difficult task because they are asked to learn a new way of thinking while, at the same time, explore their reactions to this learning as compared to a client family's reactions. It is my experience that despite the emphasis on the person in the environment most students learn only a rudimentary level of systemic thinking in their other classes.

When students enter a social work class to learn systemic family therapy, they are a self-select group, interested and curious about working with families. They have some information and expectations (the grapevine works wonderfully in college communities). They have heard that they will learn as peers and that they will learn something different about themselves and how to think about their clients. Often, they are skeptical. Will this class really be any different than any of the others they have taken? Will their knowledge base and thoughts really be heard and respected? Can they share with each other and learn from each other even if no one is 'converted'? There is one other element. These students are generally in their second and final year of Social Work School so they bring with them a certain amount of skepticism. They are 'war weary' and somewhat wizened. They want to be inspired and challenged, but they do not believe that this truly will happen; perhaps they hope it will not, for they are often anxious to just finish school.

As the class members bring their history, expectations, and anxiety to the class so does the family bring the same elements with them to treatment. As the family sits in the therapy office during the first session, they too may be skeptical. Can the therapist help us? Will our ideas be heard and respected? The family interfaces with external systems such as work, school, and religious, social and cultural groups. They learn of the world through newspapers and watching television. Their performance is appraised and judged, not unlike the students, by society, and they must learn to support each other through the joys and challenges of life.

Though this may be a new class, the students have a sense of connectedness with each other, like a family, since they have been together for at least one year. This connectedness is in the sharing of experiences of school, field work and negotiations with faculty and administration. They are excited and stimulated by their new ideas and new awareness of their personal and professional expansion. Sometimes what they learn in school and in their placements is consistent, but many times they are contradictory.

The family has had generations of connectedness (the common history that they share) and boundary setting to define themselves. As family members conduct their day to day activities they must process new information and adjust their behaviors to maintain their boundaries and their familiar level of interpersonal tension.

Both students and family members risk their sense of belonging and their familiar balance when they try on new thinking and behaviors that do not fit the structure in which they are used to living. Both groups work, at least initially, to maintain the integrity that they know and trust (e.g., their homeostatic balance). Their boundaries continue to define them as a separate and distinct unit in spite of whatever the dysfunction or need that holds or brings them together. Both the family entering therapy and the social work class will change their homeostatic balance and the texture of their relationships as they begin the new learning experience, or they will reject the opportunity to grow and change. It is the desire to grow, to change and to take risks that becomes the most important point of commonality for the healthy family and the productive class.

First and Second Order Change in the Class and the Treatment Family

The commonality shared by social work students and families in treatment is that they both want something to change. They have both come to a new situation for change, but with slightly different perspectives. Students choose to go to school and place themselves in a situation involving change and discomfort. The family, on the other hand, feels discomfort and then comes to therapy. Although wanting change, both resist or question it and, conversely, work to preserve their present structure. Students and treatment families want to feel more comfortable in their life situations and more in control. Yet they both want to do the minimum work and suffer the least amount of pain in the course of the change.

How then does a family change? When tension and anxiety take a family beyond its existing resources some form of change will occur. First order change happens when the family adds or subtracts behaviors within its familiar pattern. This decreases the tension but does not truly change the way the family members interact. Second order change alters the pattern of interaction and response between family members in a way that enables new patterns to emerge. Second order change is in the risk taking which changes the boundaries of all family members and their actions and reactions to and with each other (Watzlawick, Weakland & Fisch, 1974). The impetus for either change may be precipitated by broken rules (e.g., through telling worries to an outsider that brings outside intervention into the family); through appropriate developmental stages that challenge a family's sense of togetherness and require new responses from the family system, or through unexpected crisis, such as unemployment or illness.

An example of 1st order change might be what is commonly known as the geographical cure. The geographical cure is used by almost all families as a way of reducing tension and strife. The family member who is in conflict with the family may reduce the amount of contact in order to avoid strife. This reduction can be brief or long term. It appears to everyone as though the family has solved the problem. If, during this period of reduced contact, both the family and its members hold onto their blame, then when contact is resumed, the conflict will reappear as if there had been no break. Second order change might be illustrated by the same family member who upon reducing the amount of contact with the family comes to understand and accept her or his contribution to the conflict and is able to choose behaviors and responses that do not perpetuate that role in the old conflict. The new behavior may change the organization of the family, so that when the person returns to the family, the other members can relate to one another without being drawn into the old, predictable traps and reactive responses.

Students change in similar ways. Students learn and use information in one of three ways. They can disregard the new information totally; they can take in information that adds to their knowledge store but does not become a working part of their repertoire; or, they can use the new information to reorganize their thinking patterns. Students have a pressing need for new information that will help them feel they are moving into the professional world with good tools and adequate information. They have a sense of their own competence from past experience and a stronger sense of incompetence from their extended position of "student." What they know and what has worked for them has been challenged, questioned, augmented, and sometimes outrightly negated and denied. They must accommodate to the school's powerful hierarchy so they can maneuver through the system with their own integrity and well-being remaining intact. Students come to class looking for alternatives to take with them to the field both to help their clients and to help them feel more competent. When they are reminded or encouraged, the students tap into the competencies they have experienced. They look for ways to incorporate this with the information they have been given and continue to search for tools to deal with the complex needs of the clients and the agencies with which they work. Students are looking for ways to integrate all the information they have been given and to find tools to deal with the complex needs of their clients and agencies.

Students in this class group and the treatment family experience an imbalance and make efforts to regain a sense of control. The second year students are looking for "what to do" before they are exposed, full force, to the world of clients. Their sense of competence is shaken and they are feeling the need to fill up their "bag of tricks" (first order change) rather than to look at how they can broaden their thinking (second order change).

In a family the same parameters apply. The need to belong is strong and the rules are clear. The family may want the agency/worker to make the misbehaving member "get better" so that the family can back to 'normal,' normal being its accustomed sense of balance and, therefore, control of its functioning. If we try on something new, such as voicing a dissenting opinion from the 'family whole,' then we risk our known place in the group. How much do we risk? How far can we trust the system (class, school, family) to allow us to dissent? Families come into treatment in a state of disequilibrium, when their resources have been taxed and their alternatives for solutions have been exhausted. Similarly, families want the particular problem "fixed" (first order change) rather than explore how to expand their relational and emotional repertoire which will, ultimately, enable them to meet other crises and challenges with more creativity and less panic. However, the family, as well as students, must be willing to experience the sense of imbalance that will get them to this new place.

LEARNING REQUIRES DISSONANCE AND SAFETY

In learning systemic theory, students are challenged to think in a different way; this may precipitate a learning crisis. In crisis there is fertile ground for second order change, when the old, familiar ways no longer work or are not taken for granted. In order to maximize the second order change the environment in the classroom must be safe. An atmosphere is created that is supportive and non-threatening. The class must be a safe place for students to question and explore. It must be a safe place where they are respected for what they already know and encouraged to try new thoughts that may be incorporated with what they already know. Students are often hesitant, unsure, yet willing. While their contributions are being acknowledged they are also being challenged. Students are challenged to perceive themselves differently, challenged to perceive themselves vis-à-vis school and their agencies differently, and challenged to respect their own resources. This is a breath of fresh air, yet at the same time it creates dissonance for them. In teaching them to think systemically their linear thinking is challenged. The observations and evaluations they have been making of the dynamics and interactions of their clients take on greater dimensions. They begin feeling safe while also feeling the dissonance. How does it happen?

It is at this point that the students are made aware that these are the same reactions that families experience as they enter treatment, whether voluntarily or involuntarily. From the beginning of class, parallels are drawn between the students' experiences and the treatment family's experiences.

The class, with all new information and assignments are continually reminded to observe their responses to their assignments (e.g., how they feel doing a genogram of their family of origin) and to remember that their client families will experience similar feelings and reactions. Students are respected for their expertise about themselves; they are in a safe place; they are supported through the pain of learning new information and the confusion that comes with it. The confusion, while helping them get to their new path, is a clear signal of their exploration of new ways of thinking about and perceiving the world and each other.

Throughout the semester I help students connect their learning on three levels: their experience with their client families, the clients' experiences within their own family, and experience in their own family of origin. This works not only to clarify the implications of the students background in their therapeutic role but also to facilitate their connecting their perceptions and feelings to that of the client family's history and experience of being in therapy. Herein lies the power of this class and the experience they share as a group. The students' experience of the dissonance of new learning side by side with the sense of safety in the classroom and in the therapy helps them to understand the client-family's experience; new information can be considered, tried on and incorporated. This "safe dissonance" operates for both students and client families and, to the students surprise, it works.

AWARENESS OF THERAPIST'S OWN FAMILY

The link between the students' experiences and that of their families in their field placements is their own family of origin. Students bring with them their own experience of being in a family and recognize their experience as unique. It is clear that some students will relate class material more readily to their client population, and others will first draw upon their own family experiences. Again, this underscores that the interaction between the students' experience of their own families and their client families is what gives this class the power to create change. The structure of the class allows students to move back and forth between their two worlds as therapist and as family members themselves. This helps students recognize how difficult it is for client families to expose themselves to the therapists.

> As the class worked on a family of origin genogram, Mary stated that there were certain things she did not feel were appropriate for her to divulge in a class so she would not include them on the genogram. In recognizing her loyalty to her family of origin, she came face to face with her family's rules and secrets that were not to be shared with outsiders. Her reluctance was acknowledged, respected, and honored. From this she was able to understand how difficult it is for clients to share and expose their families.

As students make personal connections with systemic theory, they must respectfully listen to each other; they are not to comment, editorialize, or make 'brilliant insights.' It's none of their business (or mine either)!

Each step we take together reflects the steps a client family takes through the therapeutic process. Each time this is pointed out the entire class becomes increasingly sensitized to the family's position as consumer.

> In class one day Sandra become thoughtful about a family myth she had lived with as part of her family's history. The myth was that she was the one responsible for keeping the peace in her family. She always took pride in being the one family members approached for advice and caretaking. She acknowledged that if someone had directly challenged this myth she would have become defensive, not only of her family's history but of her role in that scenario. More importantly, she became aware of how families become labeled as resistant, defensive or hostile when they do not accept the social

worker's evaluation. She took this new perspective of support for the family's existing functioning back to her work setting and found that she was no longer challenging a family into defensiveness.

This freed Sandra and the client family to move forward in their work without having to abandon the family's past.

REVERBERATION OF CHANGE

Creating an environment for change is reflected throughout the hierarchy of the student's graduate school life and must not be narrowly defined as simply a classroom activity. In class we present new information and alter perceptions of currently held views. The students learn to incorporate a family systems perspective into their practice, with their supervisors, and in their agencies. This means that changes created in the classroom will have reverberations for the students in their other classes, in their field agencies, as well as with their clients. The teacher must anticipate with the students what will happen in these other systems when change is introduced. Again, this reflects what happens when family members change their positions in their families and in their communities.

At his placement agency, Ralph attempted to describe to his supervisor that the Golden family seemed not ready to move on to goals the agency had deemed appropriate for them. The case was a foster child that the agency repeatedly attempted to 'reunite' with the birth family. As often as the son was returned to his family he was shortly returned to foster care. In studying the family's history it became apparent that mothers in this family did not care directly for their children. Mrs. Golden had been raised by her maternal aunt, and her mother had been raised by her paternal grandmother. Ralph postulated that perhaps the Golden's were attempting to care for their son in the best way they could—by placing him in another home. The supervisor was able to hear his explanation but argued that the agency had to work to replace the child in the home.

The system of the worker, vis-a-vis the agency, administration, and supervisor now needs to be addressed. Through the class the students develop a perspective about their clients that may be out of synch with the perspective of their supervisor. The supervisor reflects the perspective and values of the agency. What are the risk for students voicing ideas contrary to their supervisors and agencies? The risks are the same ones that families face. To belong to a group one must follow the rules that define its specialness. Students have little power, are only temporarily part of the agency 'family,' and are in the 'child' position. Students become aware of the overt and the covert rules and the expectations of adhering to agency guidelines, and they increase their awareness of the consequences if the guidelines are not followed. The risk of students expressing a systemic interpretation of a family's problem are the potential loss of their own tenuous sense of competence and recognition, the client dropping out of therapy, a poor student evaluation, the student being labeled trouble maker or not being liked. Taking a stand different from an agency's is a vulnerable position for students.

Family members face similar risks as the students, e.g., upsetting the family, incurring someone's disapproval, a label of trouble maker. In the same way, supervisors and administrators are uncertain how to respond to and what the reverberations will be of a student's different perspective. The same is true for the family. If Mom no longer allows grandmother to make the rules about her child, she risks the familial unity she has known, however dysfunctional, as defined by their present and past history. When a family is recognized for its strengths even in the midst of the turmoil that brings them to the agency, they are able to respond in a less defensive manner. When the therapist joins with them in a safe environment (as students may do with professors or supervisors), their ability to explore their feelings and to explore alternatives is greatly enhanced.

INCORPORATING THE CHANGE

As class members share their thoughts and experiences with each other throughout the course they become less fearful and more adventuresome. They are able to explore their own hesitance or 'resistance' to trying something new. Often, students will privately share what they have tried, the results, and the impact it had on them. They need to be encouraged to share this information with the class and, in so doing, they validate the new information. This information has now become a part of the shared class experience. When students hear from the professor what works or does not work they are skeptical. Hearing from each other has greater impact and validity.

As the class progresses and students feel they have "slipped" (as students often describe the experience) from systemic back to linear thinking, they are able to recognize when the thread to the systemic thinking was lost. Often students will begin describing a family member's behavior but will catch themselves looking at causation or at a 'victim,' and realizing they have lost the systemic thread.

The treatment family walks the same path. When family members respond differently they are surprised. They begin to recognize their new responses and, with equal clarity, recognize when they seem to lose it. These changes are experienced, reacted to, and validated by the family members together and they become a part of the family's shared new reality.

AFTER THE DANCE IS OVER

As the class and the family move through their experience they continue to feel confused and challenged as well as more competent and clear about their abilities. This sounds dichotomous. The students leave the class far from being experts in family therapy. They will, however, never again view a client, a family, or themselves in the same way. Their perceptions have been challenged, their repertoires expanded, and their thinking broadened. What they take away from the class, besides theoretical knowledge and some "how to's," is a new base for collecting and organizing information from external and internal systems. While they do not have as many answers as they would like, they do have a new ability to think in a different framework, to come up with different ideas, and to pursue more varied interventions.

A family leaves treatment without all the answers but with a sense of accomplishment and mastery. They have a new reality, more problem-solving skills, and an increased sense of competency about themselves. They have expanded their repertoire to include success. The family has new tools with which to observe themselves and each other differently, and they have a greater ability to choose their responses. While they may be unsure of their gains they feel a heightened sense of their strength and ability to move through life.

CONCLUSION

New learning always creates dissonance and confusion, clarity and new options. This is true for both students and treatment families. Out of this melee of feelings comes sharper perceptions, a greater sense of connectedness, and a willingness to be in control of their being out of control (e.g., the ability to recognize when they are losing their new-found clarity and to not panic). In a safe place, it is easier to explore, to observe, to risk and to grow.

REFERENCES

Christen, D., Brown, J., Ricker, V., & Turner, J. (1989). Rethinking what it means to specialize in MFT at the master's level. *Journal of Marital & Family Therapy, 15*, 81-90.

Lippitt, R., Watson, J., & Westley, B. (1958). *The dynamics of planned change.* New York: Harcourt, Brace & Co.

Watzlawick, P., Weakland, J., & Fisch, R. (1974). *Change: Principles of problem formation and problem resolution.* New York: Norton.

Training Social Workers in Public Welfare: Some Useful Family Concepts

Mildred Flashman

This article will describe the usefulness of family systems theory and practice concepts in the training of social workers in public welfare. This three-day course, under the auspices of the Boston University School of Social Work, was developed with an awareness of the population served, the great stress under which clients and their families live and the broader socio-cultural, economic, and political context. Social workers in the various state welfare departments in which the training took place were beginning to assume the role of case manager. One goal of the training was to help as many clients as possible achieve gainful employment via education (General Equivalency Diploma GED) and training. Other public welfare services included financial assistance, provision of child and health care, housing, and parental guidance. The intent of the course was not to teach participants family therapy, but rather to emphasize a family-centered view of practice, utilizing selected family systems theory that would be relevant to their everyday work.

Prior to the beginning of the course participants had expressed an interest in discussing new ways of motivating the discouraged client who, despite many attempts, was still unemployed (even in a time of relatively high employment). In addition, there was interest in increasing the participants' skill as case managers, a role in which the workers, on the basis of their assessment, would link clients with needed resources.

The outline for the course was as follows:

Mildred Flashman, MSW, LICSW, is Associate Professor and Director, Family Therapy Certificate Program, Boston University School of Social Work, 264 Bay State Road, Boston, MA 02215. The author is a Charter Member of the American Family Therapy Association (AFTA), and Clinical Member and Approved Supervisor, American Association for Marriage and Family Therapy (AAMFT).

I. The Family

    A. Definitions and parameters of the family
    B. Types of family (open, closed, and random)
    C. Stages of family development[1]

II. Different family configurations and structures

    A. Single-parent
    B. Remarried
    C. "Re-formed" (other combinations of adults and children)
    D. Three-generational

III. The Genogram — The Family Map as a guide to understanding the family

IV. The Eco-Map

    A. Connections between families and outside systems
    B. Work in relation to family life

V. Interviewing

    A. Making the Connection
    B. Looking for Positives

The content of the course will not be discussed in detail, only the specific material that participants found most relevant. I will focus my discussion on four areas: the family and its context, the single parent mother, the use of positives, and the use of rituals to mark change.

THE FAMILY AND ITS CONTEXT

Social work has a long tradition of focusing on the family as the primary unit of attention and of attending to the context in which the family lives. Germain (1979) has stated that "social work historically has been committed to a conception of its practice based upon a person-situation formulation" (p. 3). In fact, social work's exquisite sensitivity to the relationship of people to their environment has been one of its distinguishing features in relation to other helping professions. Social work's long-time emphasis on and interest in the context in which people live their daily lives has been a precursor to the development in family therapy of the eco-map (Hartman, 1978; Hartman & Laird, 1983). Developed in

1973 for Michigan child welfare workers, this is a map that shows the relationship of client/families with various outside systems (see Figure 1). In constructing a picture that clearly depicts the nature of these relationships, labelling them as strong, tenuous, or conflicted, the worker, together with the client, can quickly make an assessment highlighting existing support systems — in extended family, friendship networks, neighborhood, churches, and human service agencies. The map serves also to identify gaps in needed services as well as conflictual relationships between caregivers in the different parts of the network. Welfare workers, as well as their clients, were often overwhelmed by the chaos in the lives of the family and by the many interconnections between clients and other systems. The eco-map was a most useful device for helping them organize a great deal of information about clients' connections with both natural and more formal networks. Thus, the eco-map was a concrete tool in lending clarity to case managers for assessing, developing, and coordinating resources for clients and their families. For a detailed description of the many uses of the eco-map, see Hartman and Laird (1983).

Figure 2 illustrates an eco-map completed by one of the participants in class. Jan Brown is a single mother, separated for 3 years from her husband, Bill. She has not heard from him in over a year. There are four children, Liz, 12, Cathy, 10, Rob, 9, and Jack, 6. The family, on AFDC, lives in a public housing project. The social worker in the welfare department has been encouraging Jan to work towards her G.E.D. She had left school after the 10th grade. Jack, the youngest, has just started school. Jan refers to her oldest child, Liz, as being very responsible and a big help in caring for Jack. Cathy, a quiet child, is asthmatic. Rob, the older boy is doing poorly in school and has been labelled by the school as troublesome. He is an underachiever, easily distracted and hyperactive.

The family has little contact with extended family members, none with Bill's family and sporadic visits with Jan's family who live in a distant state. As the eco-map indicates, the relationship between the school and family is stressful. The teacher tells Jan that she should exert more control over Rob. Jan, in turn, believes that the school should be able to discipline him. Both the AFDC worker and the teacher think that Jan is ineffectual and inadequate. The worker also views Jan as an isolated person with little connection outside of her home.

Upon completion of the map, it became apparent that Jan was more involved outside of the family than had been evident; she was active with three other neighbors, all single mothers and good friends, in attempting to secure better play space for the children. She also talked warmly about

FIGURE 1. Eco-Map*

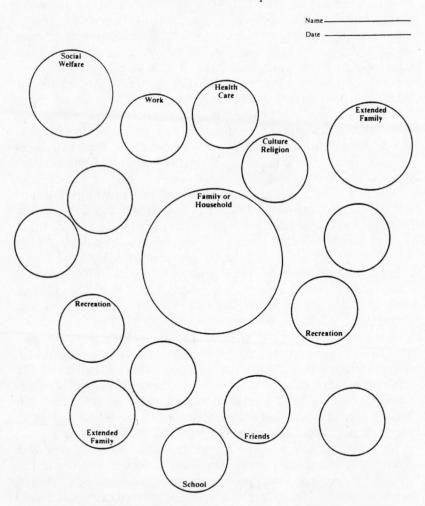

Fill in connections where they exist.
Indicate nature of connections with a descriptive word or drawing different kinds
of lines: ———————— for strong -------- for tenuous +++++++ for stressful. Draw arrows along lines to signify flow of energy, resources, etc. –> –> –>
Identify significant people and fill in empty circles as needed.

*From FAMILY-CENTERED SOCIAL WORK PRACTICE by Ann Hartman
and Joan Laird. Copyright © 1983 by The Free Press, a Division of Macmillan
Inc. Reproduced by permission of the publisher.

FIGURE 2. Eco-Map*

Name — Jan Brown

Date —

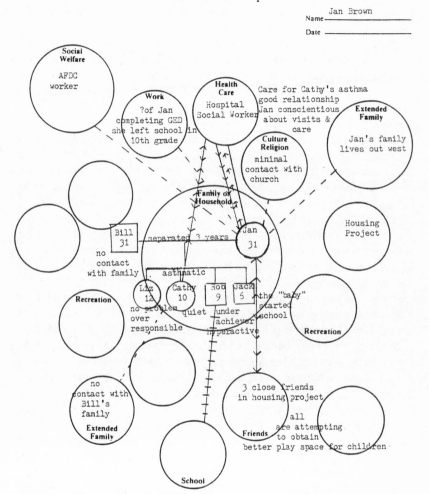

Fill in connections where they exist.

Indicate nature of connections with a descriptive word or drawing different kinds of lines: ————— for strong ———————— for tenuous +++++++ for stressful. Draw arrows along lines to signify flow of energy, resources, etc.-> -> -> Identify significant people and fill in empty circles as needed.

her relationship with the social worker in the hospital where Cathy was being followed for her asthma. As she drew the map, her perception of Jan as a mother became a more positive one.

The eco-map pointed out the lack of recreational resources for the children, especially Rob. The worker had just learned about an outreach group work program that might be helpful to Rob and planned to talk with Jan about this. With a modified view of Jan's adequacy, the worker felt more hopeful and motivated to act as Jan's advocate in relation to Rob's school.

Hartman and Laird (1983) emphasized that an important feature of the eco-map is that its construction serves as a joint venture in which both client and worker participate; it enables the client to look at herself and her family's relationships in a new way. In fact, through the map-drawing process both the worker and client may gain a new perspective. As participants reported on drawing eco-maps with clients, one worker commented that she had not realized how involved a client was on a committee in her housing project. Another client, who the worker had assumed was very isolated, was discovered to have had two very close mutually supportive friends. Hartman and Laird (1983) consider the eco-map to be both a practical and parsimonious tool. They state "The usefulness of this simple diagram becomes dramatically clear if one considers the volume of words it would take to describe the family with words alone" (p. 161). For many clients who have long been dependent on the welfare and other systems, the process of completing an eco-map can be self-empowering. A map drawn at intake, then redrawn at a later date, serves as a useful means to gauge change that may have taken place.

Imber-Black (1988; Imber-Coppersmith; 1983, 1985) presents a model for assessing and interviewing in these relationships between the family and the larger systems. She speaks of the need to reframe the term "multi-problem families" as "families with multiple agencies involved in their lives" (Imber-Coppersmith, 1983, p. 8). She suggests looking at "the meaningful system that is formed when families and larger systems come together" (p. 2), noting how the patterns that develop within the larger systems replicate the family patterns. Coalitions among multiple helpers frequently mirror coalitions in families, thus inadvertently, the helping system may often contribute to the perpetuation of many of the problems they were trying to solve. Imber-Black, as did Hartman, invites the client to take a different position as a co-observer, thus introducing new information from this perspective. This new role adds to the empowerment of the client, who as a public welfare recipient, has often felt (and been) disenfranchised, in her dependency on the system. To bring about such a shift in perception Imber-Black (1988) suggests a method of interviewing the client to obtain more information about her relationship to her outside systems. By asking questions, the client is seen as an active consumer, one whose opinion is sought and whose insight is important. Thus, the worker-client relationship is placed on a more equal level. Typical questions asked are:

- Of all the various outside helpers that your family has had over the years what did you find most helpful?

- Whom (in the family) do you think these outside involvements have helped the most?

- What do you think various representatives of larger systems have thought of your family?

- What might they tell me about working with you?

- What do you think your family's relationship with social services will be like in 5 years? (Imber-Black, 1988, pp. 94-106).

Such interviewing serves to inform the current worker (and families) about patterns of relationships with outside agencies, yielding clues as to what may or may not work and "avoids adding another helper to the system which may serve to perpetuate a dysfunctional pattern" (Imber-Black, 1988). Attending to this information is most important for case managers.

THE SINGLE-PARENT FAMILY

The largest portion of the participants' caseload consisted of single-mother families. Therefore, the discussion focused on the mother's relationship to larger systems and the issue of empowerment in relation to outside systems. Imber-Black (1989) emphasizes how some clients who are single parents become caught in a web of outside agencies. She writes:

Women may find that they are members of triangles with two or more larger systems. Here helpers often assume "parental" roles positioning the woman client in the place of a "child" whose parents are arguing over "who knows best." Such triangles often function in ways that contribute to the women's confusion and lack of confidence frequently resulting in further referrals or increased involvement of the multiple helpers thus maintaining the woman in a "one-down position." (p. 343)

Morawetz and Walker (1984) echo these thoughts when they state: "Frequently, a family will be involved with many helping systems and the relationships of these systems with each other in respect to the family will resemble the relationships of a group of angry and rivalrous relatives" (p. 333).

Course participants found it very useful to discuss ways that they might modify the deficit view of single-mother families. They recognized the ease with which the worker could slip into the role of the absent member, often inadvertently, thus confirming the mother's perception that something is missing in the family, an idea perpetuated and reinforced by many segments of society. One male participant recounted a home visit he had made to a single mother and her three sons, ages 13, 12, and 8. The mother's sense of helplessness was so pronounced that after announcing to her boys that the worker was in charge and would tell them how to behave, she then went out of the room leaving the worker to lecture to her sons (which he did). In class discussion, he thoughtfully stated that were he to repay this visit, he would not so quickly take over the authority, but would think of ways to involve (and empower) the mother. More recently family therapists and human service workers have been challenged to refute the deficit model of the woman who is a single mother and to find ways of encouraging and supporting her competence (Boyd-Franklin, 1989; Imber-Black, 1988, 1989; Imber-Coppersmith, 1985; McGoldrick, Anderson, Walsh, 1989; Morawetz and Walker, 1984; Walters, Carter, Papp, Silverstein, 1988). Among these writers there is, at the same time, recognition that single mothers need satisfying ties with extended family, church, friends, and other community supports.

Despite the severe, realistic socio-economic problems, stigma, and other stresses that many single-mother families face, their many strengths often go unnoticed. Walters (1988) reports on a study conducted that underscores the strengths that single mothers consider to be characteristic of their families and that contribute to their positive functioning. They are:

1. A single "line" of authority that simplified family decision making and decreased conflict born out of the splitting or triangulation of parents.
2. The opportunity for one parent to combine and integrate nurturing, caretaking and managerial executive functions, rather than having these functions divided by gender-defined expectations and roles.
3. Flexibility, or permeability, of generational boundaries, permitting

the expansion of opportunities for companionship between parent and children.

4. A reduced hierarchical structure with respect to household organization and management, resulting in a greater sharing of family tasks and the assumption of multiple roles for individual family members.
5. Increased expectations for the quality of family membership.
6. A heightened awareness of the family as an interdependent unit. (pp. 301-302.)

The class members were struck by what they had perceived as deficits of "minuses," such as one adult having primary responsibility for the family, which were reframed by single mothers as a "plus" or asset. Several of the workers commented on "how easy it is to see" that which is lacking in these families. Walters points the way towards opening up a different view. She states "the rejection of a deficit perspective enables the therapist to reference herself to a belief system encompassing the viability, choice, normalcy, and creative possibility in single parenting." She adds: "the pervasive influence of the deficit perspective that attaches to single parents, and the fear that their dependency, disorganization, and neediness engenders in therapists, will need to be consciously and consistently countered" p. 305.

LOOKING FOR POSITIVES

The challenge to view the single-parent family in a more positive light was discussed in another part of the course, a practice that emphasizes a *possibility* rather than a problem framework and emphasizes looking for competence rather than deficits with clients. Such a focus serves as a stimulus and motivation towards change. The importance of hope as a motivating factor in working towards change has long been part of social work philosophy and practice (Hollis & Woods, 1981; Perlman, 1957; Katz, 1975; Ripple, Alexander & Polemis, 1964;). Belief in possibilities and emphasis on positives have been underscored by many of the seminal thinkers and writers in social casework. Hollis and Woods (1981) stress the importance of "correcting the self-image [of the client] by therapeutic optimism. . . . Such optimism. . . . holds the meaning that someone believes in their possibilities, sees them better than they see themselves" (p. 309). Rapoport, as noted in Katz (1975), too, emphasizes that successful treatment predicated on the presence of two ingredients: "the element of hope and therapeutic enthusiasm" (p. 101).

In most recent years, family therapists have developed therapeutic approaches designed to help individuals, couples, and families access and expand possibilities for change through careful attention to clues of competence (Andersen, 1987; Chasin and Roth, 1989; de Shazer, 1985; Lipchik & de Shazer, 1986; O'Hanlon and Weiner-Davis, 1988; White, 1986, 1988). This treatment protocol is one that focuses "not on complaints but [rather] there is a redirection from complaints to a focus on exceptions—moments when things are going well. [Therefore], the sound of anything clients say that can possibly be interpreted as positive is emphasized" (Lipchik, 1988, p. 7). White (1988) refers to listening for and inquiring about "unique outcomes." He adds "unique outcomes provide the foundation for unique accounts or stories." Thus he invites clients to participate in the construction of a new description of the problem itself as he draws their attention to the moments that "contradict aspects of the problem-saturated description of family life" (p. 9). Chasin, Roth and Bograd (1989) speak of "converting a problem into a hope" and "activating client resources while deemphasizing current problems" (p. 122). The worker's careful attention to the language that is used by the client in the interview is cited by O'Hanlon and Weiner-Davis (1988) as useful in promoting new possibilities. For example, they state, "sometimes clients talk in such a way as to close down possibilities and give the impression that nothing can change" (p. 53). If a client should say, "I'll never get a job," when summarizing, the response of the worker might be, "*so far* you haven't gotten a job" or "you haven't gotten a job *yet*. What will be different *when* (rather than *if*) you get a job" (p. 61). Underlying this approach is the presupposition that there is hope in the possibility of achieving a desired goal. O'Hanlon and Weiner-Davis (1988) suggest that the idiomatic language that clients use in describing their interests or hobbies can be "extremely useful in developing metaphors to which they can relate easily" (p. 64).

Looking for, searching out, and tuning into new possibilities serve as potential resources to pursue further with clients. This concept brought about a positive reaction in participants. Several workers reflected that the idea of finding potential resources within the clients and their families gave them new hope and, in turn, they would be able to convey an attitude of hope to their clients. Joe was a 24-year old man who had dropped out of high school because of involvement with drugs. After several abortive treatments attempts, he had succeeded in staying drug free for over a year. He had held part-time jobs only sporadically and was on General Relief at the time of referral for employment and training. He was an avid baseball fan, talking with much animation about teams that were not favored to win, "the underdogs coming from behind to win in the last half of the ninth inning." He was especially excited by a player who had struck out twice before hitting a game-winning double. The worker referred to Joe's "coming from behind" to win after he "struck out" several times in drug rehabilitation programs and related this to job attempts, all the time talking about baseball players who "turn things around" for victories.

In some ways, this attitude served as an antidote to the discouragement of both worker and client as their behaviors often tended to mirror that of each other. The presuppositions in a worker's mind convey important messages to clients. O'Hanlon and Weiner-Davis (1988) state that "the therapist's belief about what can ultimately be achieved may be the most significant factor contributing to the client's expectation of change" (p. 45).

One worker role played an interview she had held with a client who was discouraged about the possibility of obtaining her GED. The worker then asked, "Has there ever been a time that you weren't discouraged? What would you be like?" In the client's description of what it would be like if she were "upbeat," the worker was surprised to sense a considerable shift in mood on the part of both client and worker in the simulation. As participants spent some time in small groups role playing, the atmosphere in the room changed perceptibly with much animation and raised spirits. There are important and powerful presuppositions embedded in the questions asked of clients; if, in questioning, a worker expects to find some sign of competence, she will most likely pick up some clue to the possibility of an exception to the problematic behavior. "By amplifying their descriptions of these times, clients may discover solutions that they had forgotten about or not noticed or the therapist might find clues upon which to build future solutions" (O'Hanlon and Weiner-Davis, 1988, p. 24).

Among the clients described was Mrs. Sawyer, a forty-year old single parent who found herself no longer eligible for Aid to Families with Dependent Children (AFDC) when her sixteen-year old son quit school to take a job. At the same time, a twenty-two-year old daughter, who was developmentally disabled, had become involved in a supported work program and had moved into a group residence, and an eighteen-year old pregnant daughter had moved in with her boyfriend. Mrs. Sawyer was referred to the training and employment program. Never having worked outside of her home, she felt not only her lack of any skills, but also some fear of working with other people because she didn't think she was a "good talker." In passing, Mrs. Sawyer had casually mentioned how she had talked to many teachers and helpers when her oldest daughter needed special care. In class, the worker felt that this was an area where her client had done some "successful talking." Class members suggested the worker have Mrs. Sawyer recount this experience, building on it as a focus in their future contact. Describing Mrs. Sawyer in more detail, the worker revealed that the woman had been brought up by her grandmother who had taken in boarders to support her family. This led to a discussion of the possibility of looking for competence and hidden assets in any bit of family history that a client might reveal. Stone (1988) emphasizes the importance of family stories. She states that "family stories convey the bad news, but they also offer coping strategies as well as stories that make everyone feel better" (p. 7). Such stories offer the opportunity for discovering hidden resources that can be handed down from one generation to another. Mrs. Sawyer's story about her grandmother's resourcefulness could be drawn upon as a legacy for her, something from which she could draw on for herself.

THE USE OF RITUALS TO MARK CHANGE

Rituals and their many therapeutic uses to mark change have been described in the family therapy literature. Imber-Black, Roberts, and Whiting (1988) state "In designing and implementing rituals with individuals, couples, families, or families and larger systems, five themes serve to orient the therapist's decision making: (1) membership; (2) healing; (3) identity; (4) belief expression and negotiations; and (5) celebration" (p. 50, 1988).

For social workers in public welfare agencies, discussion of the use of rituals as context and markers to acknowledge changes in daily living seemed useful, especially in relation to membership, identity, and celebration. Particularly pertinent was the idea of introducing a ritual to mark the change of status from unemployed to employed. Several workers for example, spoke of helping clients create a ritual around receipt of a first pay check. Others helped clients celebrate the receipt of their GED.

In the case of Mrs. Sawyer and her family described earlier, there were many suggestions among participants of helping the family to find a way to acknowledge and integrate all the changes that had taken place in their life: two daughters leaving home, one son leaving school and the mother's change of status. Laird (1988) points out that there is no ritual in our society to mark the important transition to being a woman whose children have grown. In fact she states that there is little to "help women mark *any* of the major transitions in their lives" (p. 8).

The transition to post childbearing is inadequately honored as the loss of children is mourned. . . . Since rites of passage are important facilitators in the definition of self in relation to society, there is clearly a need for women to reclaim, redesign, or create anew rituals that will facilitate life transitions and allow more meaningful and clear incorporation of both familial and public roles. (p. 338)

It was apparent that Mrs. Sawyer had never defined herself apart from her role as mother. Her experience is similar to that of many women from lower-income families whom Fullmer (1989) describes as primarily occupied with raising their children. He indicates that, because adults in lower-income families do not find the same satisfaction and meaning in the work they do, they tend to turn to the raising of children as "one of the richest sources of meaning" available to them (p. 558).

An increasing number of women in their 30's and 40's, with no previous work history may be referred for employment planning. No longer eligible for AFDC with their children grown, they too will need help in marking this life transition from caregiver to worker. Since "rituals function to reduce anxiety about change" and "make change manageable," the class suggested that Mrs. Sawyer and her children come together to "celebrate" the changes in the lives of all family members: in status, residence, and occupation. Several examples were suggested: the children might plan a special treat for their mother to mark the period she had cared for them; one daughter, who liked to bake, could bring a cake; all the children would exchange small gifts symbolizing their "graduation" from their previous roles. Workers shared many other examples of changes in family structure and composition that often went unnoticed in the families of their clients. There were many entries and leave-takings of long-time live-in partners, moves to different locations, children leaving and returning from placements—life events of great importance yet unacknowledged. (For more detailed description of the use of rituals, see Imber-Black et al., 1988.)

Roberts (1988) encourages the use of rituals in sessions with trainees. In referring to her work in teaching family therapists she states

Working with rituals as part of the training process allows family therapists to learn about the use of rituals in families different from their own, to examine their own ritual making capacities, and to become more aware of times when ritual might not be readily available to some families. (p. 401)

As part of the course-ending ritual, participants were asked to break into small groups and create some meaningful representations of the sessions for them. One worker drew a picture of balloons going up in the air with the word 'hope' written on them. Another person presented the instructor with a miniature sketch of a scene where the training took place.

SUMMARY

This article has described some aspects of a family systems training program for social workers in public welfare working with employment planning. Specific information about family developmental stages, structures, and different family forms were presented. The participants became familiar with tools, such as the use of the genogram and eco-map. As many public welfare clients live under difficult conditions, with a history of deficits and failures in their lives, there was emphasis on teaching workers to look for positives. The use of the eco-map and examples of ways of positively influencing attitudes of clients about themselves were judged as the most helpful parts of the course. Instilling hope in clients also gave more hope to workers who often replicated the feelings of helplessness experienced by those with whom they worked.

NOTE

1. Especially relevant material in discussing family developmental stages were the two chapters from Carter & McGoldrick, 2nd Edition, *The changing family life cycle*: "The family life cycle of poor black families" and "Lower income and professional families: A comparison of structure and life cycle process."

REFERENCES

Anderson, T. (1987). The reflecting team dialogue and meta-dialogue in clinical work, *Family Process*, *26*, 415-428.

Boyd-Franklin, N. (1989). *Black families in therapy*. New York: Guilford Press.

Carter, B., & McGoldrick, M. (Eds). (1988). *The changing family life cycle*, 2nd Edition. Boston: Allyn and Bacon.

Chasin, R., Roth, S., & Bograd, M. (1989). Action methods in systemic therapy: Dramatizing ideal futures & reformed pasts with couples. *Family Process*, *28*, 121-136.

de Shazer, S. (1985). *Keys to solution in brief therapy*. New York: W.W. Norton.

Fulmer, R. (1989). Lower-income and professional families: A comparison of structure and life cycle process. In B. Carter & M. McGoldrick (Eds.), *The changing family life cycle*, 2nd edition. Boston: Allyn & Bacon.

Germain, C. (Ed.), (1979). *Social work practice: People and environments*. New York: Columbia University Press.

Hartman, A. (1978). Diagrammatic assessment of family relationships. *Social Casework*, *59*, 465-476.

Hartman, A., and Laird, J. (1983). *Family-centered social work practice*. New York: Free Press.

Hollis, F. & Woods, M. (1981), 3rd edition. *Casework: A psychosocial therapy*. New York: Random House.

Imber-Black, E. (1988). *Families and larger systems*. New York: Guilford Press.

Imber-Black, E. (1989). Women's relationships with larger systems. In M. McGoldrick, E. Anderson, & F. Walsh (Eds.), *Women in families: A framework for family therapy*. New York: W.W. Norton.

Imber-Black, E., Roberts, J. & Whiting, R., (Eds.), (1988). *Rituals in families and family therapy*. New York: W.W. Norton.

Imber-Coppersmith, E., (1985). Families and multiple helpers: A systemic perspective. In D. Campbell & R. Draper (Eds.), *Applications of systemic family therapy*. New York: Grune & Stratton.

Imber-Coppersmith, E. (1983). The family and public service systems: An assessment method. In B. Keeney (Ed.), *Diagnosis and assessment in family therapy*. Rockville, MD: Aspen Systems.

Katz, S. (Ed.). (1975). *Creativity in social work: Selected writings of Lydia Rapoport*. Philadelphia: Temple University Press.

Laird, J. (1988). Women and ritual in family therapy. In E. Imber-Black, J. Roberts, & R. Whiting (Eds.), *Rituals in families and family therapy*. New York: W.W. Norton.

Lipchik, E. (1988). Purposeful sequences for beginning the solution-focused interview. In E. Lipchik (Ed.), *Interviewing*. Rockville, MD.: Aspen Systems.

Lipchik, E. & de Shazer, S. (1986). The purposeful interview. *Journal of Strategic and Systemic Therapies*. *5*, 88-99.

McGoldrick, M., Anderson, C., & Walsh, F. (Eds.). (1988). *Women in families: A framework for family therapy*. New York: W.W. Norton.

Morawetz, A., & Walker, G. (1984). *Brief Therapy with single-parent families*. New York: Brunner/Mazel.

O'Hanlon, W. & Wiener-Davis, M. (1988). *In search of solutions*. New York: W.W. Norton.

Perlman, H. (1957). *Social casework: A problem solving process*. Chicago: University of Chicago Press.

Ripple, L., Alexander, E. & Polemis, B. (1964). *Motivation, capacity, and opportunity*. Monograph. Chicago: University of Chicago Press.

Roberts, J. (1988). Rituals and trainees. In E. Imber-Black, J. Roberts, & R.

Whiting (Eds.), *Rituals in families and family therapy*. New York: W.W. Norton.

Stone, E. (1988). *Black sheep and kissing cousins: How our family stories shape us*. New York: Penguin Books.

Walters, M. (1988). Single parent female-headed households. In M. Walters, B. Carter, P. Papp, & O. Silverstein (Eds.), *The invisible web*. New York: Guilford Press.

Walters, M., Carter, B., Papp, P., & Silverstein, O. (1988). *The invisible web*. New York: Guilford Press.

White, M. (1986). Negative explanation, restraint, and double description: A template for family therapy. *Family Process*, *25*, 2.

White, M. (1988). The process of questioning: A therapy of literary merit. *Dulwich Centre Newsletter*, Winter.

CLINICAL

AIDS, Crack, Poverty, and Race in the African-American Community: The Need for an Ecosystemic Approach

Gillian Walker
Sippio Small

This paper will argue that AIDS in communities of color cannot be addressed without advocacy for the development of ecosystemic approaches to care which are community based and led.*

At different times in their histories both family therapy and social work have developed ecosystemic health care intervention programs, which locate the "illness" within the larger context of family, community and political system. More recently the gay community responded to the AIDS epidemic by creating holistic AIDS service delivery programs, directed and staffed by a mixture of professionals and volunteers from the community. Organizations such as Gay Men's Health Crisis and The People With AIDS Coalition empowered gay people to mobilize community resources to provide care, develop effective safer sex education programs which

---

Gillian Walker, MSW and Sippio Small, MSW, are affiliated witht he Ackerman Family Therapy Institute, 149 E. 78th Street, New York, NY 10021.

*The meaning of AIDS and crack in minority communities will be presented, followed by explanations for the type of ecosystems solutions necessary. Examples of community-based programs are provided.

spoke to the mores of the community, advocate for new treatment protocols. Furthermore they provided locations for political activism as AIDS
issues began to be seen in relation to larger issues concerning institutional-
ized homophobia and the oppression of gays. Inner city communities are
in desperate need of ecosystemic AIDS prevention and care programs that
are community based and directed. These programs would need to locate
AIDS in relation to the over-arching issues of poverty, drugs and racial
discrimination, and to provide centers where people would come together
to advocate for political change.

THE MEANING OF AIDS IN MINORITY COMMUNITIES

The threat of AIDS to both the Black and Latino communities cannot be
underestimated. The percentage of Black and Latino AIDS cases in large
Eastern cities is around 60% and Black and Latino persons diagnosed with
AIDS show substantially shorter survival times than Whites (Friedman,
1987). Most women infected with AIDS are Black or Latino and in some
areas, such as the Bronx, as many as one in forty-three babies are born
infected with the virus, ninety percent of whom are Black or Latino (Lambert 1988). An epidemic of crack and intravenous drug use accounts for
the rapid spread of AIDS in the inner cities. There are an estimated
250,000 IV drug users in New York State, at least half of whom are
infected with HIV. Crack users, estimated at well over 100,000 in New
York City alone (New York State Division of Substance Abuse Services
Report, 1989), also spread AIDS. Injectable drugs like heroin are used to
mediate the crash as the person comes off crack, and sex is used as a quick
way of obtaining crack or financing drug use. Furthermore the majority of
crack users are now women, who may become infected and will bear
children at risk for infection (New York State Division of Substance
Abuse Services Report, 1990).

In the gay community, AIDS forced an understanding that silence,
whether the silence of the closet, or silence of voices ashamed to protest
lack of government attention to a disease which was decimating the community, would mean death both of the spirit and of the body. As a result
the community organized to provide care for people with HIV infection,
prevent sexual transmission, to advocate for new treatment protocols, and
to prevent discrimination against both people with AIDS and gays. By
contrast, in communities of people of color there is an eerie silence about
AIDS while the HIV infection rate soars. Silence reflects the shame of a
disease, the silencing effects of racism, the absence of leadership at a

community level, and complex feelings about the meaning of the disease itself.

In order to create effective inner city AIDS prevention and education programs, one must understand the meaning AIDS has for the community of people of color. An article by Harlon Dalton which appeared in *Daedalus* captured many of the critical issues which shape the African-American community's response to AIDS. Dalton writes "The black community's impulse to distance itself from the epidemic is less a response to AIDS, the medical phenomenon, than a reaction to the myriad social issues that surround the disease and give it meaning. More fundamentally, it is the predictable outgrowth of the problematic relationship between the black community and the larger society, a relationship characterized by domination and subordination, mutual fear and mutual disrespect, a sense of otherness and a pervasive neglect that rarely feels benign" (Dalton, 1989, p. 205).

Dalton's analysis of the silence about AIDS in the African-American community makes several points which are crucial to planning interventions. He hypothesizes that the reluctance of the community and its political leaders to "own" AIDS is related to several key beliefs which can be summarized as follows:

(1) Since the media identifies the origin of AIDS as Africa, transmitted to the United States through Haitians, AIDS becomes just another vehicle for scapegoating people of color (Dalton, 1989).

(2) African-Americans mistrust the push from white America to "own" their AIDS problem. Furthermore, the silent spread of AIDS in the community feeds underlying fears of genocide which have been fueled by the lack of concern for the value of black lives manifest by the larger society. In the infamous Tuskegee study, conducted by the Center for Disease Control, black men were exposed to syphilis and offered no treatment so that the natural history of the disease could be followed; this has become a fable in the community which shapes belief systems about the intentions of government health officials towards blacks. That the CDC is directing AIDS initiatives does not inspire confidence among African-Americans (Dalton, 1989).

(3) AIDS has been identified as a 'gay' disease. The African-American community is strongly homophobic, a result not only of the moral teachings of the black church but further complicated by the troubled relations between black men and women. The abuses of slavery produced stereotypes of the strong black female and weak black male whose manhood was always in jeopardy. The weak male, it was feared, would ultimately be forced to abandon his woman. The gay black male becomes the em-

bodiment of these fears. A result of homophobia is that gay sex is often not acknowledged (Dalton, 1989). In the Latino community many men have regular sexual encounters with other men, but as long as they are not the receptive partner, they do not see themselves as having "homosexual" sex.

(4) Embracing AIDS means dealing with strong negative feelings towards drug users who are its major risk population. As Dalton writes, "For us, drug abuse is a curse far worse than you can imagine. Addicts prey on our neighborhoods, sell drugs to our children, steal our possessions, and rob us of hope. We despise them. We despise them because they hurt us and because they *are* us. They are a constant reminder of how close we all are to the edge. And "they" are "us" literally as well as figuratively; they are our sons and daughters, our sisters and brothers" (Dalton, 1989. p. 217).

(5) The insistence of the white community that AIDS be the priority arouses resistance in poor communities. When people are struggling with basic issues of existence, drugs, housing, malnutrition, urban violence, safety for children and families, an invisible virus does not even come near the top of the list of priorities. Dalton writes, "When we want help, white America is nowhere to be found. When, however, you decide that we need help, you are there in a flash, solution in hand. You then seek to impose that solution on us, without seeking our views, hearing our experiences, or taking account of our needs and desires. We tell you that we fear genocide and you quarrel with our use of the term. Then you try to turn our concerns back on us. "Don't you know," you ask us in an arch tone of voice, "that while you are standing on ceremony, thousands of the very people you say you care about are dying from AIDS?" Struggling to ignore the insulting implication that we are profoundly retarded or monumentally callous we respond, "Don't *you* know that they are already dying from drug overdoses, Uzis and AK-47s, joblessness, despair and societal indifference?" And, white America, you sigh and say, "What's one thing got to do with the other?" Then we sigh and wonder if you truly do not understand" (Dalton, 1989. p. 218-219).

Dalton's argument underlines the need for a holistic approach to AIDS intervention which is community-based and directed. While people with AIDS need additional services to handle illness related issues, AIDS programs should be willing to deal with all aspects of a family's life including housing, drugs, and employment. Because AIDS touches so many raw nerves, including deep suspicions of racism, intervention must be led wherever possible by people who have credibility with their clients because they are of the community. This is not easily accomplished. Even professionals of color may have to overcome suspicion that they are agents of the dominant society. For example, the African-American physician recommending AZT may encounter beliefs that the medication is poisonous, a suspicion that is not unfounded as it also has aroused controversy among gay activists. A social worker pressing the client to be tested may be seen as supporting dubious law enforcement procedures rather than actively providing help. Encouraging a woman to use safer sex may be experienced, as with other birth control measures — as a societal injunction that she is not fit to be a mother, as a way of keeping down the minority birth rate or as a means of depriving her of childbearing — the one experience that gives her life meaning, hope and dignity.

Programs must sensitize health care professionals to counter-transference issues, particularly in the area of drug use. Many professionals who have grown up in the inner city themselves have suffered from the presence of a drug user in the family and have experienced the cycles of love, hopefulness, anger and despair as family members go through the cycle of drug use and abstinence. While the stereotyping label "manipulative junkie," which professionals often use, has much truth, it also blocks out personal pain and makes it hard to hear the AIDS infected drug user's legitimate demands for help. The hostility of professionals often discourages the drug user from utilizing services which are critical to their health and that of their families.

THE ECOLOGY OF THE INNER CITY

The ecological niche promoting the spread of AIDS in the inner cities was created in the sixties and seventies as the middle classes emigrated from inner city communities leaving only the poorest of Blacks and Latinos (Inclan & Ferran, 1990). Growing up in the post War period in Harlem, the second author remembers a mixed community of the poor and middle class professionals. Community centers provided centralized care, places where a whole family was known, socialized with other families received health and dental care, had recreation programs for their children. In the seventies, cut-backs in social service budgets closed community centers. Members of the community who would normally have provided community leadership left in search of better opportunities or because they had achieved the initial goals of immigration, the upward mobility of their children. If they lived elsewhere but returned to work in their communities of origin, unlike the professionals of two generations earlier who lived in the community they served, they were not perceived as community advocates who by virtue of their professional standing had access to the dominant society but whose loyalty was primarily to their own. This loss of the middle classes from the inner cities and the resulting vacuum of leadership have had critical implications for the fight against AIDS.

Writers such as Inclan and Lemann (1990; Lemann, 1986a, 1986b) have noted that the result of all these changes was the "victory of disorganization" and the loss of the structural controls provided by family, neighborhood and religion. For African-Americans, these losses were very great indeed. Family, extended kin, religion, and community had been the very instruments through which hope had been preserved during centuries of oppression—the structures which fostered survival, connectedness, and meaning. Assaulted by the stress of urban poverty without structures which offered alternative visions, families of the inner city increasingly fell prey to alcoholism, drugs, violence between man and woman and parent and child, and the random violence within the community.

The failure of traditional structures, compounded with the denial of access to resources, prevented the acquisition of education and job skills which would provide an exit from the cycle of persistent poverty. As the cycle of poverty amplified so did the critical experience of powerlessness. And as the situation in the inner cities deteriorated so the physical isolation of inner city populations from the mainstream increased. In many cases the inner cities were a war zone where strangers entered at their peril. In systems terms the inner city was becoming a closed system in terms of real access to an outside world that could support growth, change and aspiration (Hartman & Laird, 1983). Without access to exchange of information with the outside world, the inner city becomes a classic example of an entropic system whose boundaries neither permit the importation of necessary supplies for internal health nor allow the inhabitants enough mobility to permit a meaningful exchange of information with the outside environment.

THE CRACK EPIDEMIC

What does move across the boundaries of the community are drugs and AIDS. The structure of the crack business fits the psychological and short term economic needs of a rapidly disorganizing social system, and the crack epidemic together with the growing disorganization of the community on which it preys is the perfect host environment for AIDS. Crack attracts many more women than did heroin. These women are generally of childbearing age, and they frequently bear children who are born with a positive cocaine toxicology. Both mother's and their children are at high risk for HIV infection, since women obtain crack through payment in sex and may be polydrug users, using injectable heroin to mediate the crack crash. With heroin, the percentage of females to males users was around 20%; with crack, the percentage of women users rises to 50%.*

In inner city communities AIDS often infects several family members, both parents and one or more children or in drug ridden families, several adult family members die leaving a sibling or grandparent with the burden of raising numbers of orphaned children. If the gunfire of the crack epidemic makes the urban ghettoes seem like a war zone, then the quiet destruction of whole families by the virus is as though the instrument of violence is an invisible lethal radiation or gas which has poisoned the household. The mourning process becomes more difficult for the surviving children because in many cases the word AIDS is not mentioned, the nature of the deaths shrouded in secrecy. A pervasive shame exists that has no words. A mixture of fear, shame, and anger may push the family towards concealment and secrecy, but secrecy may offer the only protection available against the reality of social ostracism, discrimination in schools against healthy children of an AIDS-infected parent, and even loss of housing. What is remarkable is that given the social risk to the family of embracing the person with AIDS, most families of drug users do continue to care for the ill person throughout the course of the illness.

In a consumer society where affluence and consumer lifestyle is everywhere advertized in the media but temptingly out of the reach of the urban poor, cocaine signifies the dream of affluence. Its earliest associations are with affluent populations. Cocaine is surrounded by myth that it is an easy road to quick cash and instant acquisition of otherwise unaffordable goods. As Jefferson Morley writes, "cocaine was the drug for those who were getting ahead and for those who could only dream of getting ahead" (Morley, 1989, p. 344).

Contrary to the myth that crack represents an underground economy for the underclass, the bulk of drug money is immediately laundered and leaves the community (Clatts, 1990). Only the "big men" in the ghettoes of East Harlem, Central Harlem, Brooklyn, Bedford Stuyvesant, South Bronx get rich off of crack, but there is always a promise of just enough cash to get large numbers of people involved in the business—as con-

---

*The typical social service solution of removing the children from drug using mothers usually backfires; the deprivation experienced by the loss of their children often increases their desire for another child.

sumers and sellers — and to encourage youngsters who are not subject to stiff legal penalties if caught, to hold and deliver the drugs (Williams, 1989).

To understand the perfect environmental fit between AIDS, crack and the inner city populations one needs to understand the crack epidemic at various levels of the system, including the psycho-pharmacological and the psychological. From a pharmacological point of view, cocaine is a highly addictive euphoriant when snorted, with still more powerful addictive properties when smoked as crack or injected (Rosecan & Spitz, 1987). Cocaine use causes neurochemical changes by significantly altering functioning in central transmitter systems, which are thought to be critically involved in mood regulation. The cocaine user moves through a cycle, from extreme euphoria and grandiosity (the high phase), through depression and anxiety (the crash phase), and back to the euphoric phase. As tolerance to the high develops, higher repeated doses result in acute tolerance to the euphoria and the development of unpleasant effects such as rebound depression, paranoia and toxicity. Addiction develops as an attempt to reverse the unpleasant effects or because of the intense craving for cocaine euphoria (Nunes & Klein, 1987). Unlike heroin where the high leads to a sense of satiation and detachment, crack users do not satiate but become activated and seek larger doses of the drug (Nunes & Rosecan, 1987).

For people living in the persistent poverty and hopelessness of the urban ghettos, the pharmacological high is reinforced at a psychological level; users experience sensations which are most probably the diametrical opposite of the feelings they experience during everyday life. During the crash these negative feelings reemerge and are exacerbated by cocaine's assault on the central nervous system. As the amount of crack used increases, alcohol, methadon, even IV heroin are necessary to mediate the crash and the unbearable after-feelings of intense anxiety and depression. Drug use may have been precipitated by these feelings but ironically it only serves to intensify them and increase the need for the drug. Heroin numbs psychic pain, while the crack high counters the depressive misery of ghetto life with a sense of activity that allows for the expression of anger.

Self medication theories of drug use point to the psychological fit between the drug of choice and the at risk populations. Since cocaine is a powerful euphoriant and triggers feelings of mobility, activism, and sexuality, it may be hypothesized that cocaine abusers may in fact be medicating an underlying depression or painful affective state elicited by traumatic losses (Khantzian, 1985; Nunes & Klein, 1987; Noone, 1979; Coleman, Kaplan & Downing, 1986). The conditions of poverty and the violence of inner city life provide a context of constant loss and mourning. Random tragedy whether from violence, poor health care, malnutrition, lead poisoning, or arson, constantly threatens the stability of families. Cocaine and more particularly crack is easily available, highly addictive, and has a symbolic aura of "luxury" producing feelings of powerfulness in the otherwise powerless and leading to the expression of anger in a population used to turning anger inward upon itself.

The experience of the urban ghetto is also one of transience and separation from traditional kin networks and support systems. Family drug research demonstrates that the children of immigrants show a high rate of addiction (Vaillant, 1966); it also suggests that the acculturation disparity between parents and children leading to diminution of parental control and losses of culture, kin systems, and support networks predisposes families to vulnerability of drug use (Scopetta, King & Szapocznik, 1977). The populations of urban ghettoes are largely immigrants—African-Americans from the South, African-Caribbeans, Latino's from Puerto Rico, Honduras, and the Dominican Republic.

The crack epidemic exacerbates the hierarchical inversions of acculturation, where parents lose control because their children belong to the dominant culture and they do not. Children are conscripted into roles in the trade because they are not subject to the stiff legal penalties for holding drugs. A job holding or delivering cocaine may give children more spending money than their unemployed parents receiving the meager allotments of food stamps and welfare. Since a teenager's clients for crack are often adults who are parents, aunts and uncles, and grandparents—the hierarchical order which seems essential for governance in families living in chaotic social situations is challenged. Since sex for drugs is the norm, young teenage women are at more than usual risk for sexually transmitted diseases and AIDS (Williams, 1989).

Statistics confirm that drug users have a far higher than normal degree of contact with their parents. The child who starts out dealing crack to bring his single parent, welfare mother the spending money she desperately needs has a powerful experience of being irreplaceable. An adult child who senses a parent's extreme vulnerability and sadness may have difficulty separating and is likely to remain enmeshed in a childlike relationship to the parents. The social conditions of urban poverty—the fragmentation of larger support systems due to immigration to the urban ghettoes—exacerbate the experience of family vulnerability, the need to stay in close physical proximity to each other even as the normal pulls of adulthood would begin a process of separation. The family experience of drug addiction, albeit often extraordinarily painful as the family endures the agitated, violent, and irresponsible behaviors common to crack users, is also an organizing one in which family members come to have fixed patterns of communication and connection around the drug use (Stanton & Todd, 1982).

Substance use is a multi-generational phenomena, (Stanton & Todd, 1982) but drug programs treat the individual and not the family leaving the children of drug users at risk for later drug use. The majority of drug users come from families where there was substance or alcohol use or where the family had suffered traumatizing loss. They in turn reproduce a family structure which places the next generation at risk. Many families include multiple substance users and the substance use of one family member may adversely affect the functioning of others. Clinical findings show that when the drug user is an older sibling, younger siblings in the family are also at risk for substance use (Coleman, 1980). Furthermore if a daughter or son has had an important caretaking role in the family or is attached to the drug using parent, that person may attempt to recreate the caretaking relationship by becoming the partner of a drug user. Before AIDS, to be the partner of a substance user was to sign on for a difficult life; now engaging in a sexual relationship with a substance user puts one at risk for AIDS.

Crack seems to appeal to women in far greater numbers than did heroin. Some researchers have speculated that crack is attractive to women because it releases the anger and frustration they feel in their daily lives (Clatts, 1990). It is possible that crack allows a woman to experience her own angry voice, much as the woman in an abusive relationship will insist on being heard by her man even if he beats her for it (Goldner, Penn, Sheinberg & Walker, in press). Many of the women who use crack have reason to be angry. Many have been mothers since early adolescence, and most are abused by the men with whom they live (Worth, 1989). The majority are the victims of incest (Kaufman & Kaufmann, 1979; Smalls, 1989). Feelings of depression, lowered self esteem, and shame, engendered by the incest experience, not only make women vulnerable to becoming substance users but also make them likely to find turning tricks an acceptable way of obtaining drugs. During a crack high, users report that the need for the drug is all consuming and precludes the thoughtfulness and preparation which condom use requires. The combination of the prevalence of HIV infection and an epidemic of sexually transmitted diseases which provide the sores and lesions through which the virus obtains entry into the blood stream is a lethal mixture for women and the children they will bear.

Drug programs have few treatment slots for women and almost none for women and their children. This absence of treatment programs for women is particularly damaging because the desperation engendered by the rapidly increasing need for cocaine together with the decrease in pleasure as cocaine use continues motivates women to seek treatment. Ernest Drucker (1990) has noticed that the desperation of the crack users may in fact make them candidates for treatment far earlier in the addiction cycle than the heroin user whose need for drugs can be relatively stable. However if the crack using woman finds no treatment slots available or finds that to enter one means losing her children to foster care, she may return to drug use to mediate feelings of despair and depression engendered by the period of abstinence.

TOWARDS CREATING SYSTEMIC SOLUTIONS

AIDS has created a health crisis that illuminates the deficiencies in the prevailing epistemology and determines the services are delivered. As we have seen in the preceding sections, neither HIV infection nor drug addiction can be separated from issues of poverty or racism. Effective prevention programs, in inner city communities should be (1) community based and led: utilizing the talents for leadership of inner city people and identifying and training talented family members to counsel others; (2) family oriented: addressing the multi-generational aspects of drugs and AIDS; (3) programmatically integrated: coordinating all services through one family case manager; (4) ecosystemic: understanding AIDS and drug use in relation to vital issues of survival in the urban ghettos. For example, safe sex education programs must also address the crucial role of childbearing in inner city communities and strengthen a mother's bonds with existing children. Women also need to be counselled with their partners around reproductive issues so that gender premises linked to traditional sexual roles can be challenged; (5) political integrated: understanding racist policies that create the environmental niche for AIDS and crack in communities of poverty and of color. As an example, founding of ecosystemic, community based and led organizations such as GMHC, energized a gay political movement as gay men understood the relationship between homophobia and the spread of AIDS.

Both social work and family therapy have in the past been notoriously apolitical, and have concentrated on becoming legitimatized as "scientific disciplines." Recent developments, though, in both professions point to ways of delivering services that are ecosystemic as opposed to classificatory (e.g., DSMIIIR), that demand political change at various levels of the system, and that are opposed to a narrow focus on either the individual or the family. A focus which draws boundaries too narrowly around individuals or families leads to treatment goals which primarily involve accommodation; an ecosystemic approach necessarily leads to the analysis of larger systems including political systems as an integral part of treatment.

In the early days of social work, the settlement house movement attempted to create holistic programs that were community based and to some extent community led. But since social work's clinical roots were in the classificatory epistemology of psychiatry, social workers began to describe social ills as diseases which could be ameliorated or cured if correctly diagnosed. As a result, in communities of people of color, social work was seen as maintaining the status quo rather than as advocating social reform. As Kenneth Clark (1981) writes in his classic *Dark Ghetto: Dilemmas of Social Power*, "Social work and philanthropy as instruments of constructive social change have so far had little impact in any of the nations urban ghettos" (p. 174). He attributes this both to the lack of indigenous leadership in social service agencies and to the prevailing epistemology of professionalized psychologists and social workers. "In their preoccupation with the individual and their insistence in reducing him to a manageable set of assumptions the disturbing and dehumanizing social realities behind his personal agony may be avoided," (p. 77). As a result, ". . . These professionals need not confront the difficult problem of the nature and origin of social injustices nor run the risks of conflict with the many vested interests which tend to perpetuate the problems of the poor and the rejected. This posture is built into the nature of their training and reinforced by their complex role as agents of the more privileged classes and the admitted and irrevocable fact of their identification with the middle classes" (p. 77).

Social work, however, has always had a thread of political activism in its sub specialty of community organization. Recently the development of ecosystemic theory has begun to provide the theoretical basis for the wedding of political aspects of social work to service delivery (Germain, C. 1979). The ecosystemic social worker became interested in the adaptive relationship between individual, family, and environment. What previously had been defined as "psychopathology" and subjected to normalizing intervention could now be viewed as attempts of systems to fit with and to maintain integrity in a problematic environment. Intervention involved an analysis of the recursive problem maintaining loops between individual problem bearer, family, environment, and culture; it might take place within or at the interface between any of these domains.

In thinking about families of people of color, a systems view would throw out Moynihan's categorizing, victim blaming "multi-problem family" concept which has become the dominant cultural narrative about people of color and of poverty. The systems thinker would be free to look at the history of the extraordinary resourcefulness of the African-American family, noting its strategies for surviving appalling oppression both psychological and economic. Adaptive strategies could be utilized in program development and intervention, for example, the power and deep loyalty of kin ties, the embracing of related and non-related children, and family members in need. One would identify coping strategies such as humor, the richness of language (Draper, 1979), the ability of the Black church to provide patterns of meaning, and locations for positive socialization in the absence of the most basic community facilities. The community of poverty then would be seen not as deficit ridden but as a rich and varied group of people with many resources who are dealing with complex social problems; a group of people with strong capacities for leadership, a tradition of hard work, and a long and deep history of mutual aid.

In the early years of family therapy, the major schools merely substituted dysfunctional family dynamics for dysfunctional individual dynamics as causal factors in the evolution of a specific mental illness. Some schools threw out the idea of mental illness and addressed problem generating sequences of communication and problem maintaining solutions as the area for therapeutic intervention. The unit of intervention was always the individual or the family and the fear was that larger units of intervention were not manageable and would dilute therapeutic effectiveness. For example, in *Problem Solving Therapy* Jay Haley (1976) argues that ". . . The most useful point of view for the therapist *is* the idea that there is sufficient variety in any situation so that some better arrangement can be made" (p. 5). While Haley discusses both the need for the therapist to intervene on behalf of the client in larger systems, and the danger of the therapist becoming an agent of social control, he is fairly representative of family therapists in narrowly defining the therapist's function.

In the nineteen sixties and early seventies a few family therapists influenced by the community psychiatry movement developed some interesting ecosystemic ideas as they designed coordinated health care programs for inner city populations. They created a model of crisis intervention therapy which utilized the resources of the clients ecosystem instead of traditional mental health facilities, and experimented with ideas like network therapy and multisystems meetings. Perhaps the most clearly articulated community based health program was E.G. Auerswald's crisis intervention program which existed for five years in the late sixties at lower Manhattan's Gouverneur Hospital.

Auerswald (1968, 1969, 1983) believed the true application of systems theory could not be confined to treating family or individual dynamics in a mental health center while the larger systems which defined family life remained unaddressed. He observed that specialization had forced individual people and families with complex social and environmental family and individual problems to shop for pieces of help. In poor communities where once the community center provided a model of holistic care, medical, social and recreational services had become totally fragmented. Clients journeyed large distances from agency to agency to obtain essential services, a Kafka-esque nightmare of waiting, filling out forms, standing in clinic and welfare lines. Services were redundant and workers only knew that small piece of the puzzle which was their domain. Auerswald's crisis intervention unit was designed to provide an antidote to the fragmentation of social service. It was to be a health care/mental health system with a single point of entry which could respond in an integrated way to all the interrelated issues—medical, social and behavioral—that created distress. Auerswald argues that the individual diagnosis or problem definition would not determine the location of care. Medical or psychiatric phenomena would be analyzed in relation to the larger context of the person's life and intervention might take place in any system which had significant impact on the problem. An important point for Auerswald was that the family/social system was the unit of care and should provide the framework for all other interventions, as opposed to family therapy being thought of as an ancillary service. A metaphor he uses is that if the therapist does not understand the context in which the symptom takes place, he may be trying to fix the fuse when in fact the power grid is down.

Auerswald emphasized the importance of the intake interview as changing both the client's and the professional's description of the problem. "The way intake is determined determines the structure of the interventive system" (Auerswald, 1983). Convening the family, or kin-friendship network was the major tool for gathering socio-cultural information about the family system. Auerswald went on to say that until network sessions were held, professionals did not see the connections between events which made up the story of which the symptom was a part, nor were they able to mobilize essential support systems. Since helping systems often maintained problematic situations, interventions to alleviate the clients problems might take the form of changing their interactions with larger helping systems. Auerswald's insights would lead to later critical inquiries into the role of larger systems in problem formation and maintenance (Imber-Black, 1988).

To be effective, the helping system must adjust to the needs in time and space of the client population. In the Gouverneur program, interdisciplinary teams made home visits, convened networks, facilitated the acquisition of any needed services even if that meant inventing services which did not exist. Reflecting ten years later on the ending of the program in the early seventies, Auerswald (1983) wrote that even though the great society programs ended, his program developed within the context of the community it served and began to shape its activities to fit needs expressed by the community. In doing so it challenged the way the dominant medical center provided pieces of service to the community (Auerswald E.H. 1983).

Despite the inherent political risks, ecosystemic programs providedp (1) sophisticated analysis of client needs, (2) the ability to formally conceptualize the family as the unit of care, (3) techniques for mobilizing the resources of social networks and extended kin systems to be care-givers and problems solvers, and (4) techniques for negotiating the interface between the multiple agencies which are often present for people of poverty.

INTEGRATED, WORKABLE, ECO-SYSTEMIC TREATMENT MODELS

The standard care situation for families where one or more members have AIDS starkly underlines the need for program's such as Auerswald's. In one family seen in an inner city hospital, fourteen workers were involved. The mother was dying of AIDS, the four year old child showed ARC symptoms, the father was on crack and heroin. Each family member had received counselling by workers in the areas which specialized in his or her medical illness or addiction. Because the mother had had various opportunistic infections during the course of HIV infection, she was known to different workers attached to specialized medical services. Father received his counselling through a methadon program and a vocational rehabilitation program. His crack use was known but not addressed since it fell outside the purview of designated programs. Mother and child were seen in the Pediatric AIDS Clinic, but the pediatrics worker had not met with the father or other family members. When mother became ill the child no longer came to pediatric clinic appointments. The pediatric staff were worried but were unable to contact the family, and did not know that mother was dying in the same hospital. When the mother died, no provisions for the child's care had been made because no one had been working with the family. The ill child remained with her father whose crack habit prevented him from providing adequate care. When pediatrics ultimately learned of mother's death, child welfare was called in and the search for a foster parent willing to take in an AIDS infected child took place. Because there was no safe and adequate living situation available, the child who had just lost her mother, had to be removed from her father and her home and hospitalized for an indefinite period of time. The sad fact is that extended family were available who might have been willing to take the child had preparations been made before mother's death, but the adoption of a child with AIDS takes counselling and preparation. By the time mother died, mother's mother, who lived in another city, and had not been informed of the gravity of the situation had just moved to a senior citizens center that did not permit children.

Imagine a different approach. The family is assigned a family case manager and an outreach worker from the community. After the case manager has gained the families trust and assessed its needs and capacities, a network meeting is convened to coordinate all social service and medical professionals involved with the family. After this meeting, all communications from medical and social services are routed to the case manager. Perhaps the case manager is a paraprofessional versed in the problems of poverty and trained in family systems work. The training of such a professional is neither long nor costly and has been done in various settings (Laird, 1979). The community worker and the case manager meet with the family often in their apartment. An AIDS health specialist visits with them on occasion to monitor the medical situation. During their visits they help mother confide her situation in other family members. The planning process begins for the little girls care should mother die, and the case manager begins a relationship with family members who indicate willingness to help provide either temporary or permanent care should father be unable to manage his drug use. Father's family is involved, and the community worker, also an ex-drug user, works with father to get him involved with a drug treatment program which will deal with crack use and perhaps acupuncture to help with detoxification. Because AIDS mothers are isolated, mother is invited to join a drop-in group of other family members who have AIDS or who have a spouse with AIDS. The drop in group helps mother deal with her shame, her helplessness as she comforts other group members. Her depression converts to activism as the group begins to advocate for needed services. The group also brings her child together with other HIV infected children, who like their mothers, are often isolated.

Models for such programs are found in Auerswald's crisis intervention program, in Gay Men's Health Crisis, and in the familiar community centers of the past which, unlike the mental health clinic, were there to meet families' needs over time, whether it be medical care, a recreation group, a place to socialize or to receive counselling around a difficult event. AIDS programs should not isolate AIDS care and HIV infection prevention information and testing services from other areas of concern, be they drugs, housing, protection from violence. Raising community consciousness about AIDS, mobilizing the community to break the silence of shame and stigma that has paralyzed collective action, would be a primary goal. Family members would be trained to talk to other members, kin and social networks about prevention and care for the ill. Women's and couples groups would focus on issues of safer sex, and reproductive decision making.

A program for women at Montefiore's Methadon Maintenance Clinic (Erik, Drucker, Worth, Chabon, Pivnick & Cochrane, 1990) has demonstrated the effectiveness of programs which contextualize issues such as AIDS. This program, designed by professionals in collaboration with women who were in the Methadon Program, provided self help groups for drug using women, many of whom were HIV infected. Methadon using women were invited as community experts, to provide information that could be used in program design. While it was acknowledged that the women were struggling with a drug problem, they were not treated as if drug use were their primary identity. Rather, they were seen as women who had experience in the community and who had aspirations for a better life for themselves and their children.

Peer counselling about HIV infection, mutual support both with AIDS issues and with drug use, led many of these women to enter detoxification programs. The professionals used their access to community resources to provide educational opportunities for women who had been previously written off by society as hopeless polydrug abusers, and to advocate for safe housing and child care. As the program evolved, the women asked for couples groups to deal directly with their male partners about issues of potential or actual infection, and for family groups to plan for the care of children when they were ill, on drugs, or should they die.

Grandparents and siblings seemed eager to come, demonstrating the ability of networks to respond to crises. The myth that men would not attend such programs was exploded when they saw that their women were enthusiastic and were getting concrete services as well as mutual support and friendship. The second author co-leads the couples group with the Women's Center's professional founder Katherine Eric; he notes that there was little need for a professional facilitator, as the group became enormously skillful at counselling each other and recruiting other families and couples to join. AIDS information was not segregated from other information; safe sex counselling was provided in couple's sessions and groups so that the gender and racial beliefs around men and women's sexual roles could be explored in an atmosphere where men and women could lend each other mutual support. A women individually counselled about safe sex, may expose herself to her partner's anger or violence if she asks him to use protection.

The success of the Woman's Center provided the idea for a program, now in its initial phase, for mothers whose babies test positive for cocaine at birth. The mothers are also either HIV infected or at high risk for infection. It is thought that heavy and continuous maternal cocaine use during pregnancy may cause long-term effects in infants born to them, similar to those caused by fetal alcohol syndrome. Problems these children may encounter include learning disabilities, hyperactivity, shortened attention span, mood swings, difficulty controlling affect, and difficulties in bonding. It is hard to tell, though, to what extent these effects are due to drug use or to the chaotic environment in which they live. Clearly, physiological difficulties will be exacerbated by a system which does not provide for continuity of care nor for the ongoing psychosocial support necessary for the families who raise these children (Drucker, 1990). Without psychosocial intervention the non-HIV infected babies who survive will be at risk for becoming the next generation of drug users.

This population of cocaine using mothers and their addicted infants was chosen for this new program to demonstrate the relationship between effective HIV prevention, the prevention of family fragmentation, the management of drug use in mothers and improved functioning in their children. Experience with drug using mothers who lose their children to the foster care system is that they tend to have replacement children. Since their partners are likely to be drug users, most often infected with HIV, it is critical for AIDS prevention to strengthen rather than weaken maternal bonds to their existing children. One drug using mother had given up nine children to foster care placement. Each time a child was removed she had another baby. The last child was HIV infected. The second author helped her regain custody of her children and advocated for adequate housing and services to reunite the family. Drug treatment programs such as the ones that had treated her over twelve years of drug use, usually minimize the importance to women of maintaining connections with family and children, while research on women shows that successful experiences of connectedness are fundamental to women's self esteem (Gilligan, Lyons & Hammer 1990). As this mother began to resume care for her children and experience success as a mother, her craving for drugs diminished.

In the program for cocaine addicted mothers outreach workers who either have been drug users or are nurturing maternal figures from the community will make the initial contact with the birth mother while the baby is being detoxified from cocaine. Under New York State law, during the babies detoxification Child Welfare Association is mandated to determine whether the baby will be placed in foster care, returned to the birth mother if she finds treatment for her addiction, or placed in the custody of a willing and suitable family member. Such decisions, which will play a critical role in the baby's future, are made in the heat of the birth crisis, by CWA workers who are overwhelmed and undertrained, and often acting on minimal information about family resources and kin systems. As a result the worker has little real assurance that the baby will be safe during the mother's involvement with drugs and treatment. Foster care with its appearance of supervision is too often seen as the least troublesome alternative, although clinicians know all too well the connection between multiple foster care experiences and later outcomes of criminality and social deviance.

If the birth mother decides to use the maternal and infant care program during her baby's detoxification, she and her family will be assigned a family case manager to advocate for the family and to arrange for necessary services over a five year period. Case management goals include arranging for kin foster care if indicated, maintaining the mother's bond with the baby even if she enters drug treatment, strengthening her relationship with her other children, helping the family mobilize resources to deal with problems that may have arisen because of drug use, facilitating the acquisition of concrete services, and coordinating larger systems involved with the family. Psycho-educational models will be used to help the family plan for the chronic relapsing aspects of drug use. Outreach workers will make contact with the birth fathers wherever possible. Simple observation of neo-natal unit waiting room suggests that many men are very involved with their families, caring for the other children while their partners visit their newborns.

In this program the mother's drug problem is conceptualized as a chronic relapsing disease, requiring ongoing availability of family support. Drug treatment is usually not conceptualized as a long term phenomenon which requires continuity of care. As a result drug users often "fail" they way through many programs rather than working with one program, in collaboration with their families, over whatever length of time it takes to remain drug free. The second author's experience in a drug free program was that when he became involved at intake with the families of the drug user, the families were able to actively support drug treatment. As a result retention improved and relapses were shorter. Families were grateful to have their own needs addressed, since they were often drained by constantly "giving" to the drug user. Attention to the family made them more willing to provide care for the user's children, which in turn enabled the mother to remain involved during the ups and downs of her drug problem.

Family members other than the index mother will be designated as "link therapists" to the program. With the case manager acting as consultant, link therapists trouble shoot and develop solutions to family problems in conjunction with the birth mother. Family members will also be trained to meet the special needs of babies born addicted to cocaine and to be sure the family can provide safe and continuous care for the children during the drug user's likely relapse. Judy Landau's model (1982) of network link therapy where family members are coached to become family problem solvers describes this useful support system (Landau, 1982).

The initial assessment meetings will be structured as network meetings attended by significant family members and other people in the family's social network, including workers dealing with other children in care, the outreach worker, and the family case manager who acts as an advocate for the family. At this meeting issues will be presented to all the agencies involved, including the Child Welfare Association, and a treatment plan hammered out. Network meetings will be convened whenever family crises or successes indicate the need for re-evaluation. The program also provides for the gradual replacement of professional family therapists with indigenous outreach workers who will be trained to become family case managers able to conduct network and family treatment sessions. Professionals will become consultants to the program as community people take over their tasks.

As in the Women's Center, support groups, multiple family groups and couples groups will be part of the ongoing program. Multiple family groups build mutual support systems and counter the fragmentation and isolation often experienced in inner city life. These groups are effective both as a way of disseminating information to other people in the community and in changing the perception of relationship with the professional from a dependant relationship to one that is essentially collaborative. The groups also provide for the emergence of natural leaders with the goal of training them to replace the professional.

The AIDS epidemic in the gay community demonstrated valuable lessons about mutual aid, about the innate skills of lay people in performing sophisticated counselling tasks and providing leadership in designing programs for their communities, about the advantages of programs which coordinate services, about the need to challenge bureaucratic procedures which prevent intelligent lay-people from having a say in policies which directly affect them. The programs discussed above, are a small way of beginning a collaboration between family therapists, social workers, and communities of poverty and of color.

REFERENCES

Alexander, B.K. & Dibb, G.S. "Opiate addicts and their parents." *Family Process*, 1975, *14*, pp. 499-514.

Auerswald, E.H. (1968). Interdisciplinary versus ecological approach. *Family Process*, 7, 202-215.

Auerswald, E.H. (1969). Cognitive development and psychopathology in the urban environment. In P.S. Graubard (Ed.), *Children against school: Education of the delinquent, disturbed, disrupted*. Chicago: Follet.

Auerswald, E.H. (1983) The gouverneur health services program: An experiment in ecosystemic community care delivery. *Family Systems Medicine, 1*, 5-24.

Clark, K. (1967). *Dark ghetto: Dilemmas of social power*. New York: Harper Torchbooks.

Clatts, M. (1990). The crack epidemic: Have we any answers? Presentation at the Family Therapy Networker Symposium, Washington, D.C.

Coleman, S.B. (1980). Incomplete mourning and addict family transactions: A theory for understanding heroin abuse. In D. Lettieri, (Ed.), *Theories of drug abuse*. Washington, D.C. National Institute on Drug Abuse, Research Monograph 30, DHHS Pub. No. (ADM) 80-967, D.C.

Coleman, S.B., Kaplan, J.D., & Downing, R.W. (1986). "Life cycle and loss: The spiritual vacuum of heroin addiction." *Family Process, 5*, 5-23.

Coleman, S.B. & Stanton, M.D. (1978). The role of death in the addict family. *Journal of Marriage and Family Counseling. 4*, 79-91.

Dalton, H. (1989). AIDS in blackface. *Daedalus, Journal of the American Acad-*

emy of Arts and Sciences, Living with AIDS: Part 2, The American Academy of Arts and Sciences, vol. 118, no. 3, Summer.

Draper, B.J. (1979). Black language as an adaptive response to a hostile environment, In C. Germain (Ed.) *Social work practice: People and environments.* New York: Columbia University Press.

Drucker, E. (1990). In Dicken's America. *The Family Networker.*

Erik, K., Drucker, E., Worth, D., Chabon, B., Pivnick, A., & Cochrane, K. (1990). The woman's center: A model peer support program for high risk IV drug and crack using women in the Bronx. Presentation to The V International AIDS Conference, Montreal, Canada.

Friedman, S.R. et al. (1987), "The AIDS Epidemic Among Blacks and Hispanics" Millbank Quarterly 65 (supp12) 477-80.

Germain, C. (Ed.) (1979). *Social work practice: People and environments.* New York: Columbia University Press.

Gilligan, C. (Ed.) (1988). *Mapping the moral domaine: A contribution of women's thinking to psychological theory and education.* Harvard University Press, Cambridge, Mass.

Gilligan, C., Lyons, N.P., Hanmer, T.J. (Ed) (1990). *Making connections: The relational worlds of adolescent girls at Emma Willard School,* Harvard University Press Cambridge Mass.

Goldner, V., Penn, P., Sheinberg, M., Walker, G. (1990) "Love and Violence: Gender Paradoxes in Volatile Relationships." *Family Process* in press.

Haley, J. (1976). *Problem Solving Therapy.* New York: Harper Torch Books.

Hartman, and Laird, J. (1983) *Family Centered Social Work Practice.* New York: The Free Press/Macmillan Inc.

Imber-Black, E. (1988). *Families and Larger Systems: A Family Guide through the Labyrinth,* The Guilford Press, New York.

Inclan, J. and Ferran, E. (1989). "Poverty, politics and family therapy: A role for systems theory" in Mirkin, M.P., *The Social and Political Contexts of Family Therapy* Boston: Allyn and Bacon.

Kaufman, E. & Kaufmann, P. (1979) "From a psychodynamic orientation to a structural family therapy approach in the treatment of drug dependency" in Kaufman E. and Kaufmann P. eds. *Family Therapy of Drug and Alcohol Abuse* New York: Gardner Press.

Khantzian, T.E.J. (1985) "The Self Medication Hypothesis of Addictive Disorders: Focus on Heroin and Cocaine Dependence." *American Journal of Psychiatry* 142; pp. 1259-1264.

Laird, J. (1979) "An Ecological Approach to Child Welfare Issues of Family Identity and Community" in Germain C. ed. *Social Work Practice: People and Environments: An Ecological Perspective.* Columbia University Press pp. 174-213.

Lambert, B. (1988, Jan 13) "Study finds Antibodies for AIDS in 1 in 61 Babies in New York City." The New York Times p1 A.

Landau, J. (1982) Therapy with Families in Cultural Transition Chapter in *Ethnic-*

ity and Family Therapy Pierce J, and McGoldrick M. eds. New York Guilford Press.

Lemann L. (1986 a) "The Origins of the Underclass. Part I," *Atlantic Monthly*, June, pp. 31-53.

Lemann, L. (1986 b) "The Origins of the Underclass. Part II," *Atlantic Monthly*, July, pp. 54-68.

Morley, Jefferson (1989, Oct. 2) "The Contradictions of Cocaine Capitalism". *The Nation* Vol 24, No. 10 pp. 341-347.

New York State Division for Substance Abuse Services Report (1990 May). New York City.

New York Times, Report of New York State Division of Substance Abuse Services (cited in Feb. 20, 1989 p. 1).

Noone, R.J. (1979) *Drug abuse behavior in relation to change in the family structure*. Paper presented at the Third Pittsburgh Family Systems Symposium, Western Psychiatric Institute and Clinic, University of Pittsburgh.

Nunes, E.V. and Klein, D. (1987) "Research Issues in Cocaine Abuse" in Spitz, H., and Rosecan, J. (eds) *Cocaine Abuse: New Directions in Treatment and Research*. Brunner Mazel, New York.

Nunes, E.V. and Rosecan, J., (1987) "Human Neurobiology of Cocaine" in Spitz, H. and Rosecan, J. *Cocaine Abuse: New Directions in Treatment and Research*. Brunner Mazel, New York 1987.

Osborne, J. (1989) "Public Health and the Politics of AIDS Prevention". *Daedalus, Journal of the American Academy of Arts and Sciences* Living With AIDS part 2 The American Academy of Arts and Sciences, vol 118, no. 3, pp. 123-145.

Rosecan, J., Spitz, H., & Gross, B., (1987) Contemporary issues in the treatment of cocaine abuse in Spitz, H. and Rosecan, J. *Cocaine Abuse: New Directions in Treatment and Research*. Brunner Mazel, New York.

Scopetta, M.A., King, O.E., & Szapocznik, J., (1977). *Relationship of acculturation, incidence of drug abuse and effective treatment of Cuban-Americans: Final report* (National Institute on Drug Abuse Contract No. 271-75-4136).

Small, S., unpublished research as Director of Family Therapy Veritas House, New York.

Stanton, M.D. (1985), "The Family and Drug Abuse, Concepts and Rationale Chapter" in T.E. Bratter and G.G. Forrest (Eds.), *Alcoholism and substance abuse New York*. New York: Free Press.

Stanton, M.D. and Todd, T. (1982). *The family therapy of drug abuse and addiction*. Guilford Press, New York.

Vaillant, G.E., (1966). "A 12-year follow-up of New York narcotic addicts: Some social and psychiatric characteristics." *Archives of General Psychiatry*, *15*, pp. 599-609.

Williams, T. (1989), *The cocaine kids*. Addison Wesley, Reading, Mass.

Worth, D. (unpublished study) (1989) "The relationship between crack using mothers and the men they live with." Women's Center of Montefiore Hospital Methadon Maintenance Program.

Home Based Work with Families: The Environmental Context of Family Intervention

Elizabeth M. Tracy
James R. McDonell

SUMMARY. This paper describes the major roles and purposes of home based work with families. The ability of the home based worker to assess and intervene directly in and on behalf of the family's environment is emphasized. Both the social environment and the physical environment of the home and neighborhood are discussed. Specific practice principles which include and make use of environmental features are presented.

The delivery of home based services has a long tradition in social work; for example, the professional services of "friendly visitors" and the work of Charity Organization Societies were carried out largely through visits and investigations in clients' neighborhoods and homes. In recent times, however, work with clients in their own homes has been a neglected area both in practice and professional training.

As social workers attained increased professional status, visits to clients' homes tended to fall into disregard and were often relegated to paraprofessional workers, such as parent aides, homemakers, or volunteer assistants. In addition, prior to the separation of financial and social services, home visits were often criticized, and rightly so, for their invasion of clients' privacy. Currently, it is primarily publicly funded social services, such as child welfare, corrections, and public health, which make use of home based intervention (Balgopal, Patchner, & Henderson, 1988). For many clients, a home based social worker is one who "takes

---

Elizabeth M. Tracy, PhD, is Assistant Professor and James R. McDonnell, DSW, is Assistant Professor at Mandel School of Applied Social Sciences, Case Western Reserve University, 2035 Abington Road, Cleveland, OH 44106.

away your children," "spies on you," or "puts you in a nursing home." No wonder, then, that home based services are met with mixed feelings both by clients and workers alike.

This is unfortunate since work with clients in their homes, neighborhoods, and other natural settings holds tremendous promise, and provides many opportunities for creative practice. This paper will explore the roles, purposes, and functions of home based work as part of family intervention. The ability of the home based worker to assess and intervene in and on behalf of the family's environment is emphasized. It is argued that a unique feature and potential of home based work is the use of the physical and social environment as both a target and resource for change. All too often services to families fail to take environmental contexts into account. Home based services, then, offer an opportunity to define and work with family problems in conceptually different ways.

BACKGROUND OF HOME BASED WORK

In recent years, home based services have re-emerged as an increasingly popular form of service delivery, particularly with families served by child welfare systems. This has been due to the growth of family based or family centered services, which view the family's relationship to the environment as the unit of attention (Hartman & Laird, 1983). The legal mandate to maintain children in their own homes (P.L. 96-272) has also hastened the expansion of home based services to preserve and strengthen families, and to prevent out of home placements of children wherever possible.

The ecosystems perspective, an emerging view in practice, is consistent with home based services. This perspective has resulted in a broader view of human problems and their context. Essentially multi-theoretical in nature, the eco-systems perspective is not a model of practice, rather, it serves as a framework for the organization of assessment data, and as a means through which the client's problem may be situationally understood (cf., Germain, 1981; Meyer, 1983; Siporin, 1980).

Appreciating the client's problem in context suggests that practitioners must understand both person and environment factors as they impinge on the nature of the problem (Germain & Gitterman, 1986). Social work's long alliance with person based theories has resulted in reliance on psychological concepts in assessing a client's problems. Less attention has been paid, in many respects, to the application of environmental theories. There are several reasons for this. First is the difficulty in developing a coherent set of environmental interventions. Person based theories, while complex, tend to derive practice techniques and strategies from a self contained set of theoretical principles. Environmental interventions, on the other hand, require knowledge of diverse theories, few of which have been developed with an eye toward clinical intervention (Meyer, 1983).

Second, environmental theories are, by and large, not as familiar to social workers as are theories of personality. While the environment clearly has been acknowledged, it is only recently that environmental theories have begun to gain place in social work practice (cf., Germain, 1983; Meyer, 1983). The specific role that environmental theories play in the development and support of human problems may be more fully appreciated by those workers exposed to their client's home environments. The home based worker is in a unique position to assess person-environment interactions, and to understand the role of social and physical factors in the development and amelioration of family problems.

PURPOSES AND FUNCTIONS OF HOME BASED WORK

Home based work, as discussed in this paper, represents both a practice technique and an approach to practice characterized by a unique set of worker values, attitudes, and skills in dealing with families and their environments (Bryce & Lloyd, 1981; Maybanks & Bryce, 1979). Perhaps the largest expansion of home based services has been in the area of placement prevention or family preservation programs. These programs are characterized by highly intensive services, delivered in the family's home, for a relatively brief period of time (Norman, 1985). The goals of these programs are to (1) protect children, (2) maintain and strengthen family bonds, (3) stabilize the crisis situation, (4) increase the family's skills and competencies, and (5) facilitate the family's use of a variety of formal and informal helping resources.

In these programs, families are approached from an empowerment perspective rather than from the view of parents or children as problematic individuals. Services are based on family needs rather than strict eligibility requirements. Caseloads are generally small so that workers can maintain maximum flexibility in meeting family needs. Most programs limit the length of involvement with the family, typically from one to six months. However, during that time period, staff are accessible to the family, often maintaining flexible hours and, in some programs, available seven days a week. Workers assume a variety of roles and tasks, providing both clinical and concrete services. In addition, extensive use is made of the natural resources of extended family, neighborhood, and community (Whittaker & Tracy, 1990).

Home based placement prevention programs serve children and families from a number of different service systems, including child welfare, mental health, and juvenile justice (cf., Heying, 1985; Szykula & Fleischman, 1985; Tavantzis, T. N., Tavantzis, M., Brown, L. G., & Rohrbaugh, M., 1985; Haapala & Kinney, 1988; Bribitzer & Verdieck, 1988). A number of theoretical models have been utilized, such as social learning, crisis intervention, cognitive/behavioral, and family systems among others (Barth, 1990). Recently, this service model has been adapted for use in preventing foster care and adoption disruption, reunifying families after children have been placed, and providing aftercare services to children leaving residential treatment.

There are a number of advantages to service delivery in the home. First, home based services are more accessible to clients, particularly those families who would not make use of or who would feel threatened by more traditional services. Some families are in such crisis or are so disorganized that getting to scheduled appointments is extremely difficult. For these hard to reach families, home based services are an effective alternative. Cancellations, no-shows and dropouts are less likely if services are delivered in the home (Kinney, Haapala, Booth, & Leavitt, 1990).

Home based services can also facilitate engagement with the family, particularly with involuntary clients. A visit to the home conveys the worker's interest in the family and can foster more cooperative, collaborative worker-client relationships. Experiencing real life events directly with the family can be a bonding experience (Balgopal et al., 1988). By going to the home, the worker demonstrates that the family is in control of what takes place (Kagan & Schlossberg, 1989). Home visits are also valuable in understanding the reality of life for families from different cultural backgrounds (Boyd-Franklin, 1989).

Assessments can be more comprehensive and accurate with information available from the home. Family members can be observed first hand interacting with one another, and environmental stressors can be directly experienced. Physical characteristics of the home can be directly observed. The strengths and limits of the family's situation can be directly confirmed and more accurately assessed. Families often feel more comfortable on their own turf, and therefore are able to relay information more reliably (Woods, 1988).

Interventions can also be designed more realistically when the worker is knowledgable about environmental factors. In addition, home based workers can be available to support, coach, model, and reinforce at critical moments for the family, such as at dinner or bedtime. New skills are also more likely to be generalized and maintained if they are practiced in the home versus solely in an office environment (Kinney et al., 1990).

Of most relevance to this paper, the delivery of services to families in their homes provides an opportunity to identify, assess, and enhance a wide range of formal and informal supportive services. By providing services in the home, the home based worker is in a good position to understand the support needs and resources of the family and to appreciate the family's ways of coping with its environment. How the environment is defined has ramifications for home based interventions.

Essentially, the environment has generally been seen as having both a social and non-social, or physical, component. The social environment consists of the range of more or less stable person to person interactions through which individual and family social development occur over time. The non-social environment, on the other hand, represents the range of inanimate objects forming the background against which social action takes place (Germain, 1983; Germain & Gitterman, 1986).

In terms of the family's social environment, home based services are better able to access all family members, even those members who initially may be reluctant to participate. In addition, home based workers can more easily make contact with natural helping networks, relatives, friends, and neighbors. In terms of the physical environment, the home based worker has first hand knowledge of a number of factors which would not be evident in office based work, including housing, space, privacy, safety, noise, pollution, etc. Changes in the physical environment can often support and reinforce other family goals.

It is important to bear in mind, however, that since the non-social environment serves as the context for social interaction, it is difficult to assess completely free from social exchange. Some elements of the physical environment have a decidedly social component. For example, although noise and air pollution are considered features of the physical environment, they are often, in part, a by-product of human interactions. Similarly, features of the physical environment may facilitate or impede social interaction. For example, a neighborhood with safe, attractive, convenient meeting places will facilitate more interactions among its members. When the non-social environment acts as a barrier to social interactions, it engenders stress and negatively affects well-being. The remainder of this article presents guidelines for assessing and intervening with the social and physical environment as a resource and aid in work with families.

HOME BASED INTERVENTION
AND THE SOCIAL ENVIRONMENT
OF THE FAMILY

The importance of social networks and social supports in mediating the stressful effects of life events has begun to greatly influence social work practice (Whittaker & Garbarino, 1983). Blythe (1983), for example, suggests that formal and informal support networks may be able to help families of ill or disabled people to cope with a disability. Similarly, involvement in religious activities is a form of support related to effective coping with stressful events (Stone, Helder, & Schneider, 1988). Family social networks play a critical role in providing emotional and material support, in serving as role models for parenting, and in linking parents with outside sources of child rearing information and advice (Powell, 1984).

The social environment of the family consists of structural and functional elements, both of which are important to assess and distinguish from one another. Structural elements include the number and types of inter-connected relationships, for example, the composition of a mother's personal social network or the range of neighborhood services available to a family. Functional elements include the quality of help provided, the perception of being supported, the functioning of relationships within the network, the manner in which supports are accessed, and the effectiveness of the social resources exchanged. Some families may be extremely isolated from sources of support, with few resources to draw upon in stressful times. For these families, structural interventions to enhance the number and types of supports may be needed. Other families may be surrounded by conflictual relationships, or may not be able to access needed resources from their network. In these situations, interventions to change the quality and functioning of supportive relationships may be needed.

Structural and functional elements can also be assessed at three different levels: (1) the social environment within the family, (2) the family's interactions with the external environment, and (3) the ways in which individual family members are differentially connected with the social environment. Assessment of the social environment can be completed via interviews, direct observation, or paper and pencil tools, such as the genogram (McGoldrick & Gerson, 1985), the eco-map (Hartman & Laird, 1983) or other network mapping techniques.

Perhaps, assessment of the social environment within the family is most familar to family practitioners (for example, see Olson, Portner, & Lavee, 1985). This includes consideration of social interactions among family members, communication patterns, formal and informal family roles, decision making styles, and internal family boundaries. Some of the questions to be addressed are: Do family members support each other? Are some individual family members particularly isolated within the family? Is the social climate of the family hostile, stressful, chaotic, or stable? Are boundaries within the family open, closed, or random?

The family's interaction with the external environment is another level of assessment. This includes both nurturant and conflict laden interactions. Some of the questions to be addressed from this perspective include: Does the family have meaningful social connections with other individuals, groups and organizations? Does the family have access to needed social resources, such as education, health care, and recreation? Is the family open to new experiences or relationships? Are social interactions generally positive or negative? Are opportunities available to share cultural, religious and other values? Are one or more family members cut off from social exchanges (Hartman & Laird, 1983)?

In order to assess the ways in which individual family members are differentially connected with the social environment, information can be gathered concerning the total size and composition of each individual's network, the extent to which network members provide different types of support, and the nature of relationships within the network can be gathered. Some areas to consider include: What are the strengths and capabilities of the social network? Do these resources seem adequate to meet the individual's needs, or are there gaps in social support needs? Are supportive relationships reciprocal, dependable, and accessible? Is the individual surrounded by a network that is negative, conflictual, or supportive of dysfunctional as opposed to functional behaviors? Is the individual capable of accessing and maintaining supportive relationships (Tracy & Whittaker, in press)?

Knowledge of the social environment at each of these levels informs home based work with families in a number of different ways. Based on the assessment of the family's social environment, appropriate goals can be established to enhance the quantity and/or quality of resources. For example, it may appear helpful to augment a family's social network, through the inclusion of volunteer helpers, such as parent aides, who can support the family's change efforts. An individual member of the family may benefit from more meaningful social connections outside the family e.g., a big brother for a school age child, an exercise class for a young mother, a support group for parents of substance abusing adolescents.

It may be helpful to include extended family, friends, and/or neighbors in home based sessions in order to enhance the functioning of the existing social network. This may involve direct training of and consultation with social network members in ways to assist the family. Or the client may be taught ways of establishing and maintaining supportive interactions with others. Sometimes, individuals require help in balancing relationships which are not reciprocal, or in dealing with others who are critical and not supportive of their efforts to change.

HOME BASED INTERVENTION AND THE PHYSICAL ENVIRONMENT OF THE FAMILY

In general, the non-social environment has been more difficult to conceptualize and to appreciate at the level of intervention than has the social environment. The difficulty stems partly from a perception of the physical environment as non-responsive. As a non-responsive component of human experience, physical objects do serve simply as a background for social interaction. More recently, however, it has been accepted that physical objects may be classified as both non-responsive and responsive in character (Wohlwill, 1983; Wohlwill & Heft, 1987).

The responsiveness of physical objects means that one may interact with an object, and that the properties of the object change as a result of the interaction. For example, a multi-colored ball will present different color surfaces as a child rotates it. Identifying the responsive nature of the physical environment has allowed for a more complete understanding of the physical world's effect on human growth and development.

In assessing the implications of the non-social environment for families, there are two essential areas to be considered: the home and the neighborhood (Garbarino, 1982; Johnson, 1987). It is important to bear in mind, however, that larger physical contexts may be relevant to individual and family functioning. A case could be made that global deforestation has potential long term effects on the overall quality of life for people. On a somewhat smaller scale, regional drought would effect the quantity and quality of foods available in local markets, driving up food costs and placing strain on a limited family budget. While these are critical issues, their sheer magnitude defies immediate application to family intervention.

The notion of home includes both physical space in which people dwell as well as the psychological meaning applied to that space (Tognoli, 1987). Most research on home environments has investigated the physical qualities of the home on the cognitive and behavioral development of children. Essentially, a rich and stimulating home environment contributes in a positive manner to children's cognitive development, overall adaptation for both children and adults, and to the development of a mutually rewarding person-environment relationship.

Both background and focal features of the home appear to be important. Background features are those which do not draw immediate perceptual attention, such as the level of noise and activity, and the size and number of rooms. Some background features can pose adverse effects; for example, high noise and activity levels interfere with the ability to attend to a task. Children growing up in such environments have difficulty acquiring auditory discrimination and visual search learning skills (Heft, 1985). The ratio of people to rooms is also important, since crowding results in loss of personal space and has been associated with a lowered sense of efficacy over environmental events (Aiello, Thompson, & Baum, 1985; Wohlwill & Heft, 1987).

Focal features are those aspects of the home which are present in awareness and typically used in daily activities, such as toys, books, television, sufficient seating, or appliances. An optimal level of stimulation is needed for individual growth and functioning. In this regard, several factors to consider include: (1) presence and accessibility of objects of a given class, such as books or toys; (2) the diversity and complexity of these objects, with diversity meaning the number of objects available, and complexity meaning the amount of information provided by any one object; and (3) responsivity, or the extent to which objects change as a result of interaction with the object. The more limited and less complex objects are in the home, the lower the level of sensory stimulation. Over time, people living in such environments develop less interest in seeking environmental input and exploration (Wohlwill, 1983; Wohlwill & Heft, 1987).

Home based workers are often able to assess background and focal features of the home by reflecting on the way they "feel" during and immediately after a session with the family. Is the home environment overstimulating or understimulating? What do the physical lay out of the rooms and furnishings convey about the people living there? Does the home invite participation and social interaction? Or do the features of the home communicate a closed system?

Intervention in the physical environment of the home would target two principal areas. First, the use of space in the home has ramifications for the family's ability to reduce interpersonal tension. Lack of private space during conflict gives little opportunity to escape a stress event. Additionally, patterns of spatial use may not recognize normal privacy needs of children and adults e.g., a teenage daughter sleeping on the livingroom couch. The home based worker can assist the family in respecting privacy for each family member, thereby helping to establish appropriate boundaries and reduce family stress.

A second area concerns the range and quality of physical objects in the home as these are likely to affect overall levels of stimulation with implications for children's cognitive and physical development. Increasing the number of objects in the home does not necessarily involve spending large sums of money. Many re-cycled and found objects can be used both to beautify the home and provide stimulating play objects, such as attractively designed magazine pictures, or clean plastic bottles filled with small colored stones.

Beyond the home is the neighborhood. Neighborhoods serve a variety of functions, including social interaction, social control, organizational ties, collective identity, and socialization (Taylor, 1982). Home based workers can assess the extent to which the family's neighborhood is fulfilling these functions. Among the physical properties which can be evaluated are aesthetic appearance, density, real and symbolic boundaries, distance, building and neighborhood size, and traffic patterns.

Physical properties of the neighborhood affect the amount of social activity which occurs. First, neighborhood population density may have both a positive and negative influence on neighbor to neighbor interactions. On the positive side, greater density increases the number of people available for social activity. On the negative side, people living in high density areas may limit social contact as a means of reducing stress. Physical distance between homes or apartments also affects social activity. Short distances increase the likelihood of running into other people who may become friends. On the other hand, the people who live the nearest are potentially the least likable because they have the greatest chance of spoiling the immediate environment by making noise, littering, and so on. Finally, levels of social activity are higher in neighborhoods which are aesthetically pleasing, free of such things as heavy vehicular traffic, graffiti, litter, abandoned buildings, and broken doors (Franck, 1980; Taylor, 1982).

The residents' perception that the neighborhood is safe and secure is another important assessment consideration. Here such features as real and symbolic barriers (fences, hedges, dead end roads) and opportunities for surveillance serve to strengthen territorial attitudes and behaviors. Proximity to major traffic arteries tends to increase neighbor's concerns about crime. Reduction of traffic flow has been associated with lower crime rates and increased outdoor social activity (Evans, 1980; Taylor, 1982; Hallman, 1984).

Two final areas of neighborhood assessment are the degree to which organizational ties and socialization are fostered. Organizational ties and rates of social participation tend to be higher in areas which have a unique physical character. The specialness associated with distinctive or homogeneous neighborhoods may bring about a greater feeling of attachment, and a desire to maintain the integrity of the neighborhood from outside threats. The degree to which the neighborhood enforces community standards of conduct, either through explicit sanctions or peer pressure, is also related to homogeneity. Since most neighborhoods are relatively homogenous, residents often share social norms and values, and adherence to accepted practices is generally understood. Extreme deviations often appear in neighborhoods which show signs of deterioration and which have highly permeable boundaries (Hallman, 1984; Wireman, 1984).

Neighborhood based interventions focus on supporting neighborhood functions, thereby facilitating individual and family adaptation. As with other forms of social work intervention, the ability to intervene at the neighborhood level depends on an assessment which takes into account the range of environmental problems impinging on a family in need. Given the interactive nature of environmental forces, though, any one intervention is likely to have multiple implications. For example, establishing block associations or neighborhood watch groups would facilitate social interaction, foster organizational ties, reduce safety concerns, as well as foster socialization activities. Similarly, working with neighborhood redevelopment and housing rehabilitation programs would tend to increase the aesthetic quality of the neighborhood, thereby increasing the likelihood of outdoor activity and neighbor to neighbor contact. The net result of intervention at the neighborhood level would be a reduction in the overall level of stress engendered by the physical surroundings. To the extent that such stress is alleviated, families may be better able to attend to concerns within the family.

IMPLICATIONS FOR SOCIAL WORK PRACTICE

Roles for Home Based Workers

As the previous discussion implies, home based workers must assume multiple and flexible roles in working with families. In addition to the direct practice roles of therapist, counselor, and teacher, home based workers often assume indirect helping roles. These may include advocate, mediator, broker, case manager, and referral agent. Teamwork and consultation with community groups may also be a needed service.

For the agency based family worker, there may be a number of obstacles to home based practice. For example, indirect services may not be reimbursable; in many agencies only direct client contact is considered a billable service so, for example, contacts with a client's landlord might not generate revenue. Some agencies may view the unit of attention in terms of an individual, and not include collateral contacts as professional social work services. In addition, agencies may be reluctant to include informal helpers due to case management and liability concerns. On the other hand, seeing the client in the natural environment gives the worker more ready access to problem relevant information and allows for the development of more immediate interventions.

For the family worker in private practice, home based work may at first seem difficult to implement. However, those in private practice have perhaps the most flexibility to adapt services to the home environment, without the administrative barriers of agency rules and regulations. Some innovative forms of privately funded casework and case management programs for the elderly and mentally ill populations are emerging which provide a full range of direct and indirect services (R. Gonzalez, personal communication, July, 1990). This may be a fee for service arrangement which is not based on the kind of service provided, rather the worker is reimbursed at an hourly rate for any contracted service, such as transportation, recreational and socialization groups, and individual and family sessions.

Dilemmas and Challenges
of Home Based Work

In addition to the administrative barriers mentioned above, there are a number of other challenges to home based work. One is attitudinal in that the home based worker cannot exert as much control over home based sessions as over office sessions. The home based worker must be flexible and must be able to overcome or deal with potential distractions, such as phone calls, in the home environment. Maintaining professional objectivity may be more difficult when a worker is exposed to more of the family's private life. There may a tendency to either over identify or distance oneself from the family. Finally, safety is often of concern to home based workers who may be in unfamiliar neighborhoods and especially in the evening. While personal concerns are realistic, often safety arrangements can be made with the family, such as having a family member meet the worker outside, or observe the worker coming and going on the street.

Another major challenge stems from the fact that social workers are not ordinarily trained in the range of environmental interventions consistent with ecologically oriented home based work. The larger dilemma of person versus environment focus has not always been adequately addressed in social work education. In order to include an ecological focus in the curriculum, students need course work both at the theoretical and practice level in person-environment interventions. In this regard, home based work with families holds implications for all components of social work education with recognition that a special set of skills, knowledge, and attitudes are needed (Whittaker, Kinney, Tracy & Booth, 1990).

Expanding the Unit of Attention

For social work, an understanding of the role of social and non-social environments on human functioning is based on the fundamental premise that person and environment interact in such a way that each shapes and influences the other toward adaptive balance. This view leads social work practice away from traditional conceptions of the unit of attention as case based, that is an individual, family, group, or community with a problem to be resolved (cf., Meyer, 1983; Siporin, 1980). Rather, attention centers on the problem itself, understood in light of the range of person and environment factors which interfere in the development of goodness of fit (Lerner, 1983). The unit of attention becomes interrelated sets of person, social-environmental, and non-social environmental factors which join to create the problem. The worker's assessment, then, seeks to continually track the changing unit of attention, analyzing person and environment characteristics in interaction (Allen-Meares & Lane, 1987).

A problem definition embracing both person and environment factors leads to an expanded arena for intervention. That is, intervention may be directed toward the person, the environment—both social and non-social—or directed toward both the person and environment at the same time (Swain & Flax, 1986). Just as there are no hard and fast rules about what form the social and physical environment should take for any given family, there is no one formula for facilitating environmental change. The specific intervention strategy depends on the individual family situation, the goals of intervention, and the form of home based service being delivered. Assessment of social and physical environmental factors must consider the family's perceptions of need, access to resources, cultural values, and physical context.

The potential of environmental intervention is that the environment becomes both a target and a resource for change (Whittaker, Schinke & Gilchrist, 1986). By facilitating or mobilizing changes in the environment, the family may be better able to maintain the change goals of professional intervention. This is the essence both of the eco-systems perspective and home based work—to not only help clients acquire new competencies in dealing with their environments, but also to help shape an environment which will be more supportive and facilitative of clients.

REFERENCES

Aiello, J., Thompson, D., & Baum A. (1985). Children, crowding, and control: Effects of environmental stress on social behavior. In J. Wohlwill & W. van Vliet (Eds.), *Habitats for children: The impacts of density*. Hillsdale, NJ: Erlbaum.

Allen-Meares, P. & Lane, B. (1987). Grounding social work practice in theory: Ecosystems. *Social Casework, 68*, 515-521.

Balgopal, P. R., Patchner, M. A., & Henderson, C. H. (1988). Home visits: An effective strategy for engaging the involuntary client. In D. H. Olson (Ed.), *Family perspectives in child and youth services*. New York: Haworth Press.

Barth, R. P. (1990). Theories guiding home-based intensive family preservation services. In J. K. Whittaker, J. Kinney, E. M. Tracy, & C. Booth (Eds.), *Reaching high-risk families: Intensive family preservation in human services*. New York: Aldine de Gruyter.

Blythe, B. J. (1983). Social support networks in health care and health promotion. In J. K. Whittaker & J. Garbarino (Eds), *Social support networks: Informal helping in the human services*. New York: Aldine.

Boyd-Franklin, N. (1989). *Black families in therapy: A multisystems approach*. New York: Guilford Press.

Bribitzer, M. P., & Verdieck, M. J. (1988). Home-based, family-centered intervention: Evaluation of a foster care prevention program. *Child Welfare, 67* (3), 255-266.

Bryce, M. & Lloyd, J. C. (Eds.). (1981). *Treating families in the home: An alternative to placement*. Springfield, IL: Charles C. Thomas.

Evans, G. (1980). General introduction. In G. Evans (Ed.), *Environmental stress*, Cambridge: Cambridge University Press.

Franck, K. (1980). Friends and strangers: The social experience of living in urban and non-urban settings. *Journal of Social Issues, 36*(3), 52-71.

Garbarino, J. (1982). *Children and families in the social environment*. New York: Aldine.

Germain, C. B. (1981). The ecological approach to people-environmental transactions. *Social Casework, 62*(6), 323-331.

Germain, C. (1983). Using social and physical environments. In A. Rosenblatt & D. Waldfogel (Eds.), *Handbook of clinical social work*. San Francisco: Josey-Bass.

Germain, C. & Gitterman, A. (1986). The life model approach to social work practice revisited. In F. Turner (Ed.), *Social work treatment* (3rd edition). New York: Free Press.

Haapala, D. A. & Kinney, J. M. (1988). Avoiding out-of-home placement of high risk status offenders through the use of intensive home-based family preservation services. *Criminal Justice and Behavior, 15*(3), 334-348.

Hallman, H. (1984). *Neighborhoods: Their place in urban life.* Beverly Hills, CA: Sage.

Hartman, A. & Laird, J. (1983). *Family-centered social work practice.* New York: Free Press.

Heft, H. (1985). High residential density and perceptual-cognitive development: An examination of the effects of crowding and noise in the home. In J. Wohlwill & W. van Vliet (Eds.), *Habitats for children: The impacts of density.* Hillsdale, NJ: Erlbaum.

Heying, K. R. (1985). Family-based, in-home services for the severely emotionally disturbed child. *Child Welfare, 64* (5), 519-527.

Johnson, L. (1987). The developmental implications of home environments. In C. Weinstein & T. David (Eds.), *Spaces for children: The built environment and child development,* New York: Plenum.

Kagan, R. & Schlossberg, S. (1989). *Families in perpetual crisis.* New York: Norton.

Kinney, J., Haapala, D., Booth, C., & Leavitt, S. (1990). The Homebuilders model. In J. K. Whittaker, J. Kinney, E. M. Tracy, & C. Booth (Eds.), *Reaching high-risk families: Intensive family preservation in human services,* New York: Aldine de Gruyter.

Lerner, R. M. (1983). A goodness of fit model person-context interaction. In D. Magnusson & V. Allen (Eds.), *Human development: An interactional perspective,* New York: Academic.

Maybanks, S., & Bryce, M. (1979). *Home-based services for children and families: Policy, practice and research.* Springfield, IL: Charles C. Thomas.

McGoldrick, M. & Gerson, R. (1985). *Genograms in family assessment.* New York: W.W. Norton.

Meyer, C. (1983). The search for coherence. In C. Meyer (Ed.), *Clinical social work in the eco-systems perspective,* New York: Columbia University Press.

Norman, A. (1985). *Keeping families together: The case for family preservation.* New York: The Edna McConnell Clark Foundation.

Olson, D. H., Portner, J. & Lavee, Y. (1985). FACES-III. Available from Family Social Science, University of Minnesota, St. Paul, Minnesota.

Powell, D. R. (1984). Family-environment relations and early child rearing: The role of social networks and neighborhoods. *Journal of Research and Development in Education, 13*(1), 1-11.

Siporin, M. (1980). Ecological systems theory in social work. *Journal of Sociology and Social Welfare, 7,* 507-532.

Stone, A. A., Helder, L., & Schneider, M. S. (1988). Coping with stressful events: Coping dimensions and issues. In L. H. Cohen (Ed.), *Life events and psychological functioning: Theoretical and methodological issues.* Newbury Park, CA: Sage.

Swain, R. L. & Flax, N. (1986). The ecological perspective: Implications for practice, process and procedure. *Arete, 11,* 17-26.

Szykula, S. & Fleischman, M. (1985). Reducing out-of-home placements of abused children: Two controlled field studies. *Child Abuse and Neglect*, *9*, 277-283.

Tavantzis, T. N., Tavantzis, M., Brown, L. G., & Rohrbaugh, M. (1985). Home-based structural family therapy for delinquents at risk of placement. In M. P. Mirkin & S. Koman (Eds.), *Handbook of adolescent and family therapy*, New York: Gardner Press.

Taylor, R. (1982). Neighborhood physical environment and stress. In G. Evans (Ed.), *Environmental stress*, Cambridge: Cambridge University Press.

Tognoli, J. (1987). Residential environments. In D. Stokels & I. Altman (Eds.), *Handbook of environmental psychology*, New York: Wiley and Sons.

Tracy, E. M. & Whittaker, J. K. (in press). The social network map: Assessing social support in clinical social work practice. *Families in Society*.

Wireman, P. (1984). *Urban neighborhoods, networks, and families*. Lexington, MA: Heath and Co.

Wohlwill, J. (1983). Physical and social environment as factors in development. In D. Magnusson & V. Allen (Eds.), *Human development: An interactional perspective*. New York: Academic.

Wohlwill, J. & Heft, H. (1987). The physical environment and the development of the child. In D. Stokels & I. Altman (Eds.), *Handbook of environmental psychology*, New York: Wiley and Sons.

Whittaker, J. K. & Garbarino, J. (1983). *Social support networks: Informal helping in the human services*. New York: Aldine.

Whittaker, J. K., Kinney, J., Tracy, E. M. & Booth C. (Eds.). (1990). *Reaching high-risk families: Intensive family preservation in human services*. New York: Aldine de Gruyter.

Whittaker, J. K., Schinke, S. P., & Gilchrist, L. D. (1986). The ecological paradigm in child, youth, and family services: Implications for policy and practice. *Social Service Review*, *60*, 483-503.

Whittaker, J. K. & Tracy, E. M. (1990). Family preservation services and education for social work practice: Stimulus and response. In J. K. Whittaker, J. Kinney, E. M. Tracy, & C. Booth (Eds.), *Reaching high-risk families: Intensive family preservation in human services*, New York: Aldine de Gruyter.

Woods, L. J. (1988). Home-based family therapy. *Social Work*, (May-June), 211-214.

Doing with Very Little:
Treatment of Homeless Substance Abusers

Insoo Kim Berg
Larry Hopwood

INTRODUCTION

The problems of the homeless population have drawn increasing attention in the past several years. Although they have always existed in this country, the homeless population in the 1980's is more diverse than that of earlier years where the stereotype was a drunken, single, middle-aged male. The homeless now include all ages; men, women, and children, temporary and chronic; black, Hispanic, and white; rural and urban (Institute of Medicine, 1988). Although ethnographic data are not as extensive for the earlier population, the current one shares with it the same problems of mental illness and drug and alcohol abuse. Mental illness and substance abuses are higher than that of the general population with estimates of 30 to 40% (Lamb, 1984) for mental illness and 20 to 45% (Wright and Knight, 1987) for substance abuse.

Substance abuse in the homeless is a growing concern. Drug abuse is combined with alcohol abuse, and in many instances, this is compounded by the co-morbidity with mental illness. Frequently it is difficult to sort out the primary problem. A proportion of the homeless attribute their loss of housing to substance abuse problems while others cite their homeless condition as a cause of their substance abuse (Institute of Medicine,

Insoo Kim Berg, MSSW is Executive Director of the Brief Family Therapy Center, 6815 West Capitol Drive, #300, Milwaukee, WI 53216. Larry Hopwood, PhD, is the Director of the Training and Research at the Center.

A preliminary report of this work was previously presented at the AFTA meeting in Colorado Springs, CO in 1989.

The authors wish to thank Brother Joel Frank, Director of the Community Meal at St. Benedict the Moor, and the many homeless individuals who patiently answered our numerous questions.

1988). In many cases, searching for a linear causal relationship is not only difficult but also not helpful.

Short term solutions have not been successful in solving long term problems. Temporary housing shelters remove the homeless from the streets but do not solve other problems which prevent them from obtaining affordable, stable housing. Without a stable residence, it is difficult for them to obtain access to needed health care to address both med!cal and mental health problems. And without tackling these issues, it is impossible for the homeless to maintain stable employment or relationships.

The standard approach to substance abuse usually involves an inpatient detox program as the first step. However, these programs have limited space and often see repeated visits by the same clients. They are successful for some but there is no way of knowing who will benefit the most. Because the problems of the homeless are not limited to the substance abuse, a simplistic solution of substance abuse treatment does not seem to work.

Despite all that has been written about the problems of the homeless substance abusers in recent years (National Institute of Alcohol Abuse and Alcoholism, 1987), very little has been written about what does work for them. One exception is William Miller (1985) who has written extensively on the importance of linking client goals with successful treatment outcome in alcohol abuse treatment programs.

This article provides a detailed description of our study. We asked the homeless what they thought would be helpful for them and then utilized this information to empower them to make changes. The simple but true social work tenet of "Start where the client is" is given lip service but is often forgotten.

BACKGROUND FOR THE STUDY

Milwaukee's homeless population is similar to that of many other major cities: a diverse mixture of age, sex, race, and educational backgrounds. The problems of homelessness are compounded by several factors typical of other cities: 980 single occupancy units lost since 1980 in the downtown redevelopment; high unemployment due to the poor economy of industrial Milwaukee: and unmet mental health problems resulting from emptying of the psychiatric institutions (Rosnow, Shaw, and Concord, 1986).

Estimates of Milwaukee's homeless population range between 2,000 and 3,000 of which 40% to 80% are faced with problems related to their alcohol and or drug use. Although woefully inadequate, various attempts to meet the needs of the homeless are in place, including the Health Care for the Homeless, emergency shelters for 700-800 people each night, and several meal programs providing 2000 meals daily.

Located within walking distance of downtown Milwaukee, the meal program provided at St. Benedict the Moor serves approximately 500 meals, 6 nights a week and is a central meeting point for the homeless who use the services provided by the nearby social agencies. Unlike most other programs that are used sporadically, this meal program provides a consistent opportunity for the homeless to remain in contact with their friends and staff at St. Benedict's.

Because approximately two-thirds of the participants in the meal program continue to use the services over a 6 month period, the staff at St. Benedict's were able to form some impressions over time about the problems of the homeless with the existing substance abuse treatment programs in the community: the goals and protocols of these programs do not fit the lifestyle of the homeless; the goal of total abstinence is particularly realistic. The homeless themselves reported that many of the existing treatment programs were too confining, overemphasized the need to talk with others, and were not interested in the special problems of the homeless. Faced with the growing frustration over the difficulty in accessing currently existing treatment facilities, the authors wanted to talk with the homeless directly and explore alternative approaches that may adapt more closely to their needs and circumstance.

SOLUTION FOCUSED APPROACH

Since 1978 the treatment team at the Brief Family Therapy Center (a non-profit research and training institution located in Milwaukee) has been developing an innovative treatment approach called Solution-Focused Brief Therapy which is extensively described in the literature (de Shazer, 1985, 1988). Based on the General Systems Theory of Von Bertalanffy (1981), and applying the tradition of Ericksonian clinical practice (Zeig, 1982; O'Hanlon, 1987), the model pays detailed attention to patterns around exceptions to problems as clues to solving them. The model further postulates that the pattern of activities solutions is considerably around different than the patterns that center around problematic situations. Therefore, enlarging and increasing the frequency of solution patterns are the key clinical activities by the worker. For example, it is believed that finding out what the homeless do to cut down, refrain, or abstain from drug or alcohol use and getting them to repeat this, increases the frequency of abstinency and lengthens the period of sobriety. This approach is more helpful to the clients than focusing on their failures. It is also assumed that since they do have exceptions to the substance abuse on their own, even though they do not see them as small successes, therapeutic intervention is directed at increasing the frequency of exceptions to problems.

When clients either report that they have no exceptions or are unable to remember under what circumstances their life was even a little better, the use of "miracle questions" directs clients toward a hypothetical solution to problems in their future, thus focusing their attention on changing behavioral, cognitive, or emotional components of their drug or alcohol use. Future focus is emphasized when clients are asked the following question: "Suppose there is a miracle while you are sleeping and your problem with drug and alcohol (or homelessness) is solved. What would you be noticing different the next morning that will tell you that there has been a miracle?", or "What will your friends notice different about you that will tell them something is different about you?", "What will they see you do different then?"

STUDY, SITES, AND PARTICIPANTS

The study was performed primarily at the St. Benedict the Moor meal program and at various sites which form the circuit in the daily life of the individual homeless adult (homeless families and single mothers are more likely to use other services):

- Guest House Over-night Shelter
- Drop-In Center Day-time Shelter
- Guest House Health Care Center
- St. Benedict the Moor Health Care Center

At these sites initial contacts were made to engage the participants to serve as volunteer consultants on the problems of drug and alcohol use in their population. Whenever possible, sessions were held at the Brief Family Therapy Center and videotaped with the participant's consent. None of the participants were paid.

The criteria for participant selection were very broad: multiple unsuccessful attempts at managing their drug use, admission of a substance abuse problem, and willingness to be consultants to the study.

Questions were asked to obtain basic demographic data such as age, education, marital and family status, and housing information. The history of their drug and alcohol use and treatment attempts was traced. Then a series of questions was asked to determine how the participant had already tried to solve their problems, what had worked or not worked, and what they had found most helpful. The following questions were asked to learn more about the participant's perception of what in a program would be helpful to them:

1. What would you say was most helpful about your treatment experience?
2. What was least helpful about your treatment experience?
3. If you could plan your own treatment program, what would you put into it?
   What would you leave out?
4. When was the most recent time you did not use drug/alcohol?
5. WHEN and HOW do you decide it is time to COOL IT?
6. HOW do you manage not to use during this "cooling" period?
7. When you decide to "cool it" again, what will it take?
8. What will others notice different about you when you are using a little bit less drug/alcohol?
9. What difference will it make in your life then?

STUDY FINDINGS AND OBSERVATIONS

Thirty six people who admitted to a substance abuse problem agreed to volunteer to be interviewed in depth. They included 29 black males, 3 white males, 1 American-Indian male, 2 American-Indian females, and 1 Hispanic male; their ages ranged from 22 to 67 years. Our sample, predominantly single black males, is representative of those people using the meal program at St. Ben's.

Demographic Information

The following is the summary of the participants' profiles:

- The length of homelessness ranged from 3 months to 20 years.
- All have had multiple job histories; some were very skilled. About one-third of the men worked currently now and then.
- About one-quarter could be diagnosed as mentally ill. Some were currently on anti-psychotic medication, and receive psychiatric treatment.
- Approximately three-quarters have had misdemeanor charges or convictions and most reported having been in jail or on probation sometime in their life.

- About one-half of the men and both of the women maintained some form of contact with family members, such as, brother, aunt, sister, mother, and frequently their children. One man who recently became homeless said his children did not know that he was homeless; he was too ashamed to tell them.

Drug and Alcohol Problems

- All alcohol/drug abusers had varying periods of abstinence, either through treatment or on their own; some for a few days at a time, others for up to 8 months, or even 3 years. One man said he always made sure to be sober on Sundays when he called his mother.
- All were "self-medicators." That is, being chronic users, all had considerable knowledge of how alcohol/drug affects their body and knew how to bring on the desired "highs"; what brand names to use when and what dosage was best to bring on the best high.

Treatment Experience

- Out of the 36 participants all but 2 have been in a treatment program and all reported having tried home remedies to stop or cut down their use, including self administered detox or "cold turkey" with varying degrees of successes.
- Unsuccessful formal treatment attempts ranged from 1 to over 100 times, including detox, half-way houses, in-patient 28 day treatment, repeated use of Antabuse, out-patient, AA, NA, CA, "rap groups." Most reported being drug-free while in jail. All were quite familiar with conventional alcohol and drug treatment philosophy.
- About three-quarters reported that the in-patient setting (even for detox) was too confining and they felt "cooped up." They disliked the structured regime of schedules.
- 90% reported they found the information about the physiological effects of alcohol use helpful.
- The majority (85%) found the group therapy sessions not helpful. "It's a lot of bullshit." Some reported having lied, saying what the counselors wanted to hear. Some (45%) reported feeling intimidated by the lack of ability to articulate in group sessions.
- Questions about their past successes had a tremendous impact on them: jobs, promotions, family life, how they were able to help others, how their mothers were proud of them, when they had a place of their own, good clothes, money they once had, happy times in their lives, and so on. When discussing these, they visibly

changed; they became more confident, smiled more, and sat up straight.

- Responses to the "miracle question" were clinically significant. Those who were able to imagine a different reality after "the miracle" looked different even momentarily. They smiled, looked up, made eye contact with the interviewer, and sat up straight. Those who were unable to imagine a different life for themselves tended to be depressed and generally saw no hope for getting better. Approximately 80% were able to describe "miracle pictures," about 10% were unable to imagine their life being different in any way, and the rest required considerable help in imagining a changed view of themselves.

Goals and Desires

- The majority (80%) indicated that what they found most helpful was the positive encouragement, having someone who has "confidence" in them and treats "me as a real person."
- About 75% of those who currently used alcohol/drug reported no intention of stopping alcohol use but all wanted to "cut down" on alcohol use. However, almost all wanted to quit drugs. Five thought that using "pot" prevented them from getting into hard drugs.

General Impressions

Contrary to the myths about the homeless, the group as a whole is quite resourceful, independent minded, and wants the same things as everybody else: to be valued, respected, and to have freedom of choice. All wanted a place of their own, a relationship with a lady or a man, nice clothes, and money in their pockets.

CASE EXAMPLE

Herbert, a shy, soft-spoken, 32 year old black homeless man, has been a poly-drug and alcohol abuser since junior high school days. He said he used "whatever I can get my hands on" but primarily cocaine and alcohol. He had a long history of psychiatric hospitalizations with a diagnosis of paranoid schizophrenia, and several suicide attempts.

Even though he asked for "some sort of program" during our initial session he was not sure if he really wanted to give up his drug or alcohol use.

Appreciating his honesty about not being sure what he wanted to do, the interviewer asked what might be the "good reason" for doing drugs. He was taken aback, surprised at the question. Then he said he never thought about "good reasons"; he just did drugs out of habit. He composed himself and then responded:

Herbert: When I'm on the street and shoot dope I feel like somebody.
Worker: I'm sure you do. What else would you say is the good reason for doing drugs?
Herbert: Most of the time I do drugs when I don't give a damn.
(Later)
Worker: Now let's look at the good reason for not doing drugs.
Herbert: Well, I will have more money, more respect from my sister and my father, and will have things I want. But most of all, I will have my health.
Worker: So looking at both sides, how will you decide which way you want to go?
Herbert: It doesn't seem like a hard question, but it is. It is hard for me to know which way to go.
Worker: How will you know which is the right way to go?
Herbert: It seem like a right and wrong thing. But I always do the wrong thing.

At this point, Herbert talked about his latest thought of shooting himself but decided against it since he couldn't do it. "I'm not even going to think about it. But I read somewhere that drug use is a suicide."

When asked about the most recent time he was able to stay drug free, he mentioned that about a year ago he was clean for 7 months. Surprised to hear this, the worker asked how he managed to be drug free for so long. He minimized it saying that it was while he was "in a program," which he left after 7 months. When the worker persisted with this 7 months of abstinence even though there were temptations around, he became surprised at his own success.

When asked about what will help him get back to doing what is "good for you," he related his long-time dream of going to school. In fact, he attended a technical school for about a year and earned fairly good grades. He was staying with his brother at the time but wore out the goodwill. What will help you get back into school? He decided it will help him to have a place of his own; it is very difficult to concentrate on his studies while staying at the shelter at night and wandering the streets during the day.

Since his SSI payment was usually used to buy drugs as soon as he got the check, he did not have enough money for a security deposit for a room of his own, another dream. Herbert has never had his own place.

Through various channels, our project gathered enough money for a security deposit for a tiny apartment for Herbert. This was about a month after we first met. Herbert became more coherent; his drug use decreased considerably but he continued with alcohol use; he started to take a bus on his own, which he had been too fearful to do before. In order to supplement his SSI, he started to work odd jobs. It was touching to see him trying to learn to cook, pay utility bills, and do laundry, all for the first time in his life.

Follow-up a year later: Herbert's episodic drug use continued while his alcohol use increased to the point that he could not maintain his apartment. He eventually gave it up and entered a half-way house again where he has been for 4 months at the time of this writing. His drug and alcohol use stopped completely, but more importantly he has become much more assertive, and more outgoing. He is healthy looking and has developed a relationship with a young woman, a first for him. His next goal is to get his own apartment again, and eventually live with his "lady friend" which he has never done before. He still has a dream to go to school someday.

DISCUSSION

Although this study was not designed as a treatment project, and therefore we do not have follow-up data on all the participants, the information provided in response to our questions and the several extended case histories allow us to make some tentative conclusions and suggestions. This study confirms the results of others in regards to the complex nature of the problems of the homelessness: drug and alcohol abuse, recent and chronic homelessness, mental illness, poverty, and lack of social connectedness. However, sitting and listening to the homeless in their setting, instead of making them fill out long questionnaires, produced some additional useful information. Even though most had tried and failed in traditional substance abuse programs, all had significant periods of abstinence. They could also be sober for days if they had a particular purpose or goal for staying sober, such as pressure from lady friends, someone they felt close to, and family obligations. One man said he made sure he was sober on the days he looked for shoes or clothes from various clothing banks. Only after he secured these necessities, did he resume drinking.

We realize that our findings cannot be generalized to a larger population since our study is limited by the small sample size. Nevertheless, it produced a different picture of the homeless than other studies. Instead of being totally helpless and not caring about their condition, the individuals we interviewed were for the most part quite resourceful in surviving under very difficult conditions. What they want is not too different from what mainstream Americans want in terms of physical comfort, material possessions, and personal sense of satisfaction. Like most of us they want to be valued, be respected, and have freedom of choice. The absence of means to provide the latter may be one of the major reasons most treatment approaches have failed. In light of our findings, we would like to suggest that the following be considered by anyone designing programs for the homeless.

1. Need for a better fit between the client and the program.

One of the most striking and early lessons we learned is the need to be flexible and "loose," to find the fit between the culture of the program and that of the client. For a simple example, it is better to have the treatment facility near where the homeless "hang out." One man in our study said that he once had a high fever and had to walk 7 miles to the public medical facility.

The treatment program and procedures must be adaptable to the clients' goals. For example, distinction must be made between those who want to abstain from alcohol and drug use entirely and those who just want to "cool it." When the homeless feel "railroaded" into signing up for a program, they are likely to fail.

2. Access to treatment services at all levels.

The treatment program should be readily accessible to clients, not only geographically but also culturally. Clients feel out of place and out of sorts when they are not dressed well, do not comprehend the professional jargon, and do not feel comfortable in the setting.

Therefore, mixing of the middle-class, white professional or working class clients who have jobs and a supportive family with the homeless population in the in-patient setting, for example, will create feelings of inferiority, inadequacy, and reluctance to stick to the program.

3. Long-term view of success. It takes numerous small pieces put together to make a success.

CONCLUSION

Many participants in this study have been able to obtain the various "pieces of the pie" at different times: they abstained from drug and alcohol or at best moderated its use; they have held jobs; they have been in and out of temporary housing, and have had relationships with opposite sex sometime in their lives. However, frustration came when they sought help in putting it all together. Most traditional programs fail to give them credit for what they are already doing that is successful. Instead, they are pushed into programs that do not fit their needs or desires at that time. Forcing a program on the homeless does not work. They become discouraged and drop out. Even worse is that the gains they have made are lost when this happens.

They say they need help getting the next little piece of their "miracle picture." Many times they have a pretty good idea of what the picture will eventually look like and how much time it will take to complete the picture. We must accept their logic: for instance, why give up the pleasure of drugs and alcohol use until there is something else to make them feel good.

Programs must be prepared to help the homeless when they are ready to take the next small step, no matter what that might be, and continually support small measures of success. Therefore, programs must be comprehensive to include elements of housing, employment, mental health, in addition to drug and alcohol treatment. In addition, these must be intensive enough and sustained to stay with the clients no matter what course they take.

REFERENCES

de Shazer, S. (1988). *Clues: Investigating solutions in brief therapy.* New York: W. W. Norton.

de Shazer, S. (1985). *Keys to solutions In brief therapy.* New York: W. W. Norton.

Institute of Medicine (1988). *Homeless, health and human needs.* Washington, D.C.: National Academy Press.

Lamb, R., (1984). *The homeless mentally ill.* Washington, D.C.: American Psychiatric Association.

Miller, W. (1985). Motivation for treatment: A Review with special emphasis on alcoholism. *Psychological Bulletin, 98*, (1), 84-107.

National Institute of Alcohol Abuse and Alcoholism (1987). *Alcohol health and research world. Special report.* Washington, D.C.: U.S. Government Printing Office.

O'Hanlon, W. O. (1987). *Taproots.* New York, W. W. Norton.

Rosnow, M., Shaw, T., & Concord, C. (1986). Listening to the homeless: A study of homeless mentally ill persons in Milwaukee, *Psychological Rehabilitation Journal, 9* (4), 64-77.

Wright, J. & Knight, J. (1987). *Alcohol abuse in the national health care for the homeless client population.* Washington, D.C.: U.S. Department of Health and Human Services.

Von Bertalanffy, L. (1981). *A systems view of man,* Boulder, Colo.: Westview Press.

Zeig, Jeffrey, (1982). *Ericksonian approaches to hypnosis and psychotherapy.* New York: Brunner/Mazel.

The Community Residence as a Family: In the Name of the Father

Barbara Lou Fenby

From cruising the chronically mentally ill up and down the Rhine river, to housing them in asylums, to moving them to public shelters, the implicit public policy emphasis regarding care of the mentally ill has been on social control and exclusion of these people who are different (Foucault, 1973). In the 1970's when American public policy moved toward having mentally ill people live in group homes, there was an explicit definition of such homes as family-style living. This paper explores the ways in which bureaucratically designated community living situations can be considered both as families and as mechanism of social control. By examining the social construct of the community residence in this way, we are engaged in a deconstruction which illustrates how a single term like community residence can hide oppositions and power differences (Alcoff, 1989). Since social workers have based their profession on humanist values like fairness, it is important for them to understand that their daily social practice depends on such social constructs which cloak power and repressiveness from their awareness. It is fitting that a deconstructive awareness should enter social work through family therapy, since the theoreticians in this area have shown an openness to linguistic and non-positivist epistemologies (Anderson and Goolishian, 1988; Efran, Lukens, and Lukens, 1988).

IN THE HOSPITAL

When they live in the state hospitals, people who have mental illness are assigned a

---

Barbara Lou Fenby is a Social Worker in a management position with the Massachusetts Department of Mental Health at Medford State Hospital. Correspondence may be addressed to: Barbara Lou Fenby, Medfield State Hospital, 45 Hospital Road, West Hall, Medfield, MA 02052.

minority status . . . that does not have the right to autonomy, and can live on grafted onto the world of reason. Madness is childhood. Everything at the Retreat [asylum] is organized so that the insane are transformed into minors. (Foucault, 1973, p. 252)

As Foucault has explained, the asylums were constituted as simulated families around the mad/child, whereby "signs and attitudes" (1973, p. 254) of the family are recreated through the minor patient and the adult caretakers who embody Reason as assumed by the Father. In the community care of clients today, these same elements appear. The client continues to have an assigned status as dependent and child, and the caretakers assume the mantle of adulthood, carrying out the state's Reasonable mandate, in the Name of the Father.

Father in this abstraction is the symbol of patriarchal rule, which is the rule of the entitled, generally white, always wealthy, and mostly male power structure that dominates in the Western world. This power structure maintains itself by excluding those who are different. Females, the poor, and minorities are routinely relegated to the margins of society, although a few who act like the dominant male may be accepted. As disabled people, the chronically mentally ill also fall into the category of those who are excluded from power, but they traditionally have served as token children cared for through the benevolent Father. The role of the clients living in community residences must be considered against the backdrop of their assigned roles as powerless children in a patriarchial society.

TO THE COMMUNITY RESIDENCE

Liberal social workers take pride in the development of community residences, which in the early seventies were the alternatives to continuing care in the state hospitals. Because there were no clear conceptual models for this alternative housing, and because caretakers had few expectations for these long-term disabled psychiatric patients, the group homes of this era originally were designed as custodial institutions in the community. The residences were planned to be lifelong or at best transitional homes for those being moved from the state hospitals into the communities. These residences still exist in the community, although the original population of longterm hospitalized clients has changed over the years as many of these clients exceeded original predictions and have moved to less restrictive settings. These early group homes often have eight to twelve residents who live together by reason of bureaucratic expedience. Beds are filled with the next available state hospital discharge, the main criteria being the chronicity and gender of the prospective resident. Gradually the population changed; the elderly clients, socialized into the complaint patient role, now are joined by the young chronic clients. These under-forty-year-olds retain vestigial identities as functioning adults, lack lengthy hospitalization and socialization into the patient role, and have a resistance to custodial care models.

In some areas the large group homes have been augmented by apartment programs for two to six clients. Whether staffed or staff supported, these apartments are filled in the same manner as the group homes, by client need as determined by a governmental or quasi-governmental organization. Client choice about these options is generally secondary to the provider's need to keep beds filled and the state's need to retain control of people whose psychiatric symptoms could be problematic to the community. As a recent article on rehabilitation of the chronically mentally ill points out, "the history of mental health services show a persistent disregard for the needs of persons with psychiatric disability to chose housing alternatives consistent with their personal desires or goals" (Blanch, Carling, and Ridgway, 1988, p. 47).

THE FAMILY AS THE PATTERN
FOR COMMUNITY RESIDENCES

Since community residences are recent creations, how do the clients, the staff, and the general public understand what they are? Making sense of our world, and creating meaning for new social structures is common-place in the postmodern era which is characterized by rapid social change, immediate media coverage, and a sense of impending panic. To make sense of the world, individuals construct meanings of what they experience and frequently use a metaphor for "understanding and experiencing one kind of thing in terms of another" (Lakoff and Johnson, 1980, p. 5).

Community residences were initially conceptual adjuncts to the state hospitals, but their placement in residential neighborhoods required that they be framed in a way that was more acceptable to the community. This led to the framing of community residences as family-style living groups. The use of the metaphor of the family was bolstered by the prevailing philosophy of client normalization and treatment in the least restrictive environment. There were not many other ways to understand this structured communal living, and during this era social workers and the social sciences were becoming re-enchanted with the family as a concept and a subject for study. Thus "family" became a metaphor for group homes. Any metaphorical composition allows people to focus on the similarities between objects while it hides the dissimilarities (Lakoff and Johnson, 1980, p. 10). In encouraging the metaphor of the group home as a family, the issues of social control and bureaucratic institutional format are hidden from view, while other aspects of collaboration and intersubjective creation of meaning are emphasized.

LIZZY AND THE MOVE

The following section explores how family theory about shared history, myths, and rituals help inform social workers about community residences. A myth is a language, linked by "insistence and repetition" (Barthes, 1972, p. 11) that is significant for a group. The development of a shared history and the emergence of a myth and accompanying ritual is exemplified in this story of a community residence for geriatric state hospital clients.

> A group of patients had been moved to a halfway house on the grounds of the state hospital, and from this group eight were selected to move to a new community residence about twenty miles away. The Director of the Community Residence decided with the clients that they could have a pet, so they instituted a "Cat-Scan" and went to animal shelters looking for their pet until they found Lizzy. Meanwhile, in preparation for the move, a series of group meetings was held to discuss moving with these people who had been in the hospital for a combined total of over 200 years, with an average of about 30 years. The prospective community residents were frightened, had little experience with mutual concern, and no recent experience in self determination. As the time for moving drew near, each person became more psychotic-appearing and less able to communicate verbally about feelings. Suddenly one of the least stable clients focused on Lizzy and how she could be moved. The group drew together around plans for Lizzy: how she could be prepared for the move, would she need to be medicated, would she need to be caged, who would carry her, what if she didn't like it, what if she ran away. As the symbol for the group, Lizzy's adjustment was critical for each of the eight residents who followed Lizzy's example in settling in the new house and gradually exploring the neighborhood. After five years, Lizzy remains a symbol of good adjustment, and the clients vie for caring for her and for one another.

"Lizzy and The Move" is a part of the shared history of the house, and new residents are told the story and old residents enjoy the retelling. This bit of shared history has elements of a creation myth, it enshrines a set of beliefs about the past and about how the group emerged from the State

Hospital. Myths like "Lizzy" are important because they help people to "understand the world as continuous" and to "escape the terror of a world that appears indifferent" to individuals' needs (Harries, 1990).

MYTHS

This particular myth offers hope for new residents who are in transition from the State Hospital into the community. It ties the new group member to the success of the past move and allows them to realize that some of the "old ones" from the myth are still alive and in the community. This enhances the prestige of the longterm residents and helps solidify the group. Lest anyone not be cognizant of the myth, the livingroom is dominated by a large stylized graphic painting of Lizzy with the original housemembers. Since newcomers to the house generally ask about the vivid painting, prospective employees and residents have an opportunity to hear the myth as they enter the residence. The ritual re-telling of the myth further bind the residents together.

A social worker dealing individually with a client in this residence without knowing this myth is handicapped in much the same way that a family therapist is hampered by not understanding the family myths. Imagine, for example, the befuddlement of the client and therapist when the group begins to scapegoat a new resident who locks the cat out or shoos her from the living room. The shared history of the residence and the mythical presence of the cat that define the incident are missing for outsiders. At the same time, the residential staff through their understanding of the myths, and by being part of the group that repeats and believes in these narratives, are in a position to use the created family myths to leverage change. Therapy clients who live in community residences can be better understood against the background of their bureaucratically designated living group. Just as therapists are eager to meet with families to influence change, therapists might wish to consider meeting with and at the community residence which can exert mythical pressures on their clients. In extending the metaphor of family to community residences, one must include the staff and the residents as part of the family.

The community residence as a social structure can itself be seen as mythic. This is quite consistent with the traditional family, which in itself can be viewed as a myth. Each individual's understanding of the metaphor of family is experiential (Lakoff and Johnson, 1980, p. 19) based on experience in one's own family and based on the media image of the family. The media image of the family is not a real family, but the Ozzie and Harriet image becomes a concept of the family, to be copied by other media copies of the family, which are simulacra of the family. The simulacra is a copy, removed in time, space, or texture from the original. This copy spawns its own copies which beget more copies, and all purport to be the original. Indeed they are original, which causes confusion about what or whether there is *any* original, since the first original can change as a result of its copies. The simulacra become more real than real families, and play into the individual's experiential understanding of the metaphor of family. It is this complicated metaphor that all residents and staff bring with them to the community residence. The created community-residence-as-a-family is an image of an image of a family, in which the "mother is the simulacrum of territoriality, and the father as the simulacrum of the despotic law" (Deleuze and Guattari, 1986, p. 269). In community residences, the mother/residential director is on site and defines day to day situations, the father/the Law is distant and embodied in a state bureaucrat or agency director. It is probably not coincidental that four of the best-run community residences I have known over the years have been run by women, three of whom were trained as nurses. Since nurses are trained to exercise authority on behalf of the powerful doctor, they fit comfortably into the Deleuze and Guattari concept of the family as well as into the bureaucratic desires of a community residence.

In the same way that the image of the family impacts on the community residence, simultaneously the media image of the community residence impacts on each community residence. The influence of the simulacra of the community residence occurs as the media image removed several times from the original becomes the pattern for the recent original. It is within this amalgam of images that the client lives; a social worker cannot understand a community residence client without appreciating the context of these diverse pressures which contribute to the family of the community residence.

Two examples of such pressure show the impact on the individual clients. Each community residence is created with some bureaucratic objective, which is not necessarily explicated. The more clearly it can be stated, the more coordinated the residence can be in activities directed toward a specific goal. For example, a traditional community residence of eight clients had a vaguely stated goal of providing a home and helping the residents avoid further hospitalization. Client improvement was incidental to client and community safety. The tone of the house was slightly dispairing, since nothing much was expected of either staff or clients. Residents who were newly placed at this home often created problems—such as refusing to accede to what few requests were made. This was defined as part of the clients' illness; eventually the clients gave up challenging and sat quietly in front of the television set with a minimum of group interaction. In this house most of the communication was between the individual client and the staff, mirroring the interaction between young dependent children and parents. While the excuse might be offered that the residents in this home related in dependent fashion because of their illness, the unanimity of response among new residents points to an adaptation to the existing family culture.

A more recent group home, also for eight people from the state hospital, was established as a residence for those who were mentally ill with a substance abuse problem. This is a very difficult population of clients, and the rules of the house were explicit about no caffeine, attendance at five Alcoholics Anonymous or Narcotics Anonymous meetings a week, and participation in an Outward Bound style adventure program. Behavioral expectations and timelines to leave the program were set for all residents prior to entry, all staff were trained in substance abuse relapse, and some recovering alcoholics were on staff. These recovering staff members attended AA meetings with the clients and provided role models for clients. All staff took part in camping trips, where some clients were more experienced and comfortable than some of the staff. In this program clients also challenged the norms, only they organized collectively against the caffeine ban. Staff defined the challenge as healthy and responded with nonpunitive discussion, setting a tone in which norms were clear but could be questioned. The resulting interaction between residents is high in the program, and the relationship between residents and staff, while at times intense, is not dependent. This is a very different style of relating from the previously discussed residence. Community residences differ as much as families differ, and a unified concept of "community residence" would handicap a social worker dealing with a resident at any house. Just as social workers were encouraged to look beyond the individual to the family, now they must look beyond the client with severe mental illness to her/his family at the community residence.

THE EXTENDED FAMILY

Returning to the metaphor of family that each individual carries to the residence, it is useful to explore a ring of expectation that comes from the family members of the residents. These families have been through the tragedy of labelling one member as mentally ill and have had to adjust their behavior accordingly. Subsequently, they have their own definition of what it means to be a family. Many of them are parents who are in their sixties and older who desire that their children be safe and cared for perpetually, often with the sub-expectation that they become normal, at least in behavior. Not surprisingly, family members desire that the community residence meet their experiential metaphor of family and behave as an extension of their own family's protectiveness and pressure for normality. This extended family for each resident forms a network of in-law style expectations for the group residence as an achieved family. To imagine the impact of this, think of seven or eight in-law relationships impinging simultaneously on a family unit.

Institutions like mental hospitals or nursing homes have negative connotations, and families often struggle with the burden of feeling that they abandoned a relative who must be placed. Families experience the guilty relief of being free from the burden of daily care, but they also question their own motives in placing a relative in an institution (Harbin, 1988). To define the community residence as such an institution would be to court those same feelings of guilt and ambivalence. To define the community residence as a different family—for example, a group of roommates— minimizes the trauma of placement in longterm care. For the family separating from the resident, such a definition maintains the illusion of normalcy, but this illusion places another layer of demand on the residence.

> Mark, in his early twenties, had a psychotic break at college, was admitted to the state hospital, and then went to a community residence. The family defined this move as similar to being at school, and they were distressed at the appearance and behavior of Mark's housemates. As they had when he was at school they took him home on weekends and did his laundry. Five years later, Mark was still frozen in his family's definition of him as a college student while the family and residential staff were blatantly hostile to one another. Mark had no relationships inside the community residence and was frequently scapegoated by the other residents.

The family members of the community residents place pressure on the residents and the staff to behave in accordance with their own personal metaphorical interpretation of family. Since many staff members are young, without in-laws but with experience in distancing their own parents, staff respond to the resident's parents by labelling them "interfering" or "intrusive." This sets up loyalty conflicts for the resident, whose confusion can easily be identified by either side as evidence of mental illness. When an evaluation of the mental status of a resident is requested, social workers should be aware of these tensions which can cause the resident distress and symptoms which may mimic but may not be mental illness.

THE FAMILY RECREATED
IN THE COMMUNITY RESIDENCE

Inside the community residence, all the interactions known as "family dynamics" can be seen in operation. For example, sibling rivalry is frequently evident, particularly in seeking staff attention.

Lester knew that individual support generally was given to residents experiencing difficulty. When he saw the other client meeting alone with the house manager, Lester became demanding of the manager's attention. The manager, a woman in her late thirties with adolescent children of her own, had to set limits on Lester's intrusiveness after he: interrupted the meeting with the other resident, demanded the manager's time with his own story of a crisis that paralleled the "favored" resident's problem, blocked the manager's passage in the hallway, and physically prevented her from leaving the site.

In this case, the manager's own life experience led her to the interpretation of the behavior as rivalry. She responded with limit setting intervention that de-escalated the increasingly disruptive behavior. In similar crises, I have seen younger staff, in their early twenties and not far removed from their own family rivalries, define such behavior as mental illness and respond with a crisis intervention. The training of junior staff by social workers with expertise in family dynamics may help the staff develop insight into their own family constellations. Training may well improve staff ability to interpret daily events in the residence and to construct them as normal, even if conflictive, behavior.

There are some characteristics within the group home that would make it difficult for any adult to feel comfortable and there are some characteristics that bind the clients together. The former are not within the control of the residents, and are organizational factors that keep the adult in the client status of minor child, dependent on the Father. Such factors include the sharing of bedrooms with other residents and being overseen by house staff who frequently are much younger. The factors that bind the residents are often within their control and include such things as celebrating holidays or selecting an activity.

THE RULE OF THE FATHER

Many community residences are older homes with large double bedrooms. Two or three residents may share these rooms, with assignments of new roommates as the beds become vacant. There are not many adults who would choose to share a living space, especially a bedroom, with someone they did not know. The privacy of the resident is severely limited, and no conscious attention is given to the problems of personal modesty standards or the possible choice of the client to masturbate. Modesty and sexuality are not given any consideration in planning for these residents, since their dependent status leads to the denial of their personal desires, just as adults deny these desires of children. Even in newly constructed community residences double rooms are still included. The rationales are that the clients will learn to relate to one another and that they will not be able to isolate themselves and fantasize. A closer look at the rationales indicates that control of the resident is given precedence over client autonomy, so that the paternalistic needs of the Father keep the child dependent.

Staff for the community residences are generally drawn from young adults who have finished or are working on their undergraduate training. They are often idealistic, caring people who are considering professional careers in human service. Some have unresolved personal issues that draw them to working with disadvantaged people, so that they might enhance their own fragile self esteem. The residents are frequently older, sometimes old enough to be the parents and grandparents of the caretaking staff. The reversal of the age/dominance pattern creates problems, as the residents resist being told what to do by staff they view as children or as siblings. Children or siblings acting in the name of the Father disrupt the usual pattern of age expectations.

RITUALS AND ROUTINE

Predictable routine provides security (Giddens, 1984, p. 50) and community residences are highly structured so that residents might remain stable. Routines include times to get up, times to go to bed, times to eat; other routines include where clients are permitted to be, where they put their belongings, how they can organize their rooms. Routines are ways of organizing time and space. While total institutions have rules regulating space/time, community residences allow more flexibility. Any power relationship involves a dialectic between the powerful and less powerful participant, between the autonomy of one and the dependence of the other. The unpowerful dependent still is a personal agent and could "act otherwise" than comply with what is expected (Giddens, 1979, p. 148). In the community, where the mentally ill individual's civil rights are strongly protected and where there is a verbalization of client determination, the mentally ill person frequently has the opportunity to act otherwise, i.e., choose to disobey or confront the rules.

"Acting otherwise," however, has its drawbacks. While assertion and autonomy are prized in theory, inside of some families and some community residences, to act otherwise is to risk being defined as mentally ill. Since progressing from the community residence to independent living requires appearing not mentally ill, and since appearing mentally ill places the client at risk for return to the hospital, routine is generally adhered to with few sustained, overt protests.

What does happen over time is that the original routine gradually erodes to accommodate the needs of the individual clients. Without confronting the routine directly, clients—like children—find ways of getting around what is expected. They manage to secure dispensations for themselves, and the longer they stay in a residence, the more individualized their routine is.

> Isabella did not like living in the community residence, and considered herself better educated and of a better social class than her fellow residents. She minimized contact with them in the early evening hours by going to bed, but would wake up at 5 a.m. to cook breakfast for herself and the staff. While technically not within the rules, this behavior was not seen as pathological but as "just Isabella." When other clients attempted similar variations on the sleeping schedule, it was defined as a sleep disturbance and as pathological.

To the degree that residents have social skills, they can work within the structure of the residence to flex the routine according to their desires. This raises difficulties, since if the staff encourages social skill development by the clients, then the clients will be better able to negotiate the routine. For some staff it is more comfortable to keep the routine rigid by minimizing the social skills development of the clients. In this regard, the family of the community residence is not unlike families who cannot move beyond the stage of childhood compliance and into the adolescence of the younger family members.

Rituals such as holiday meals or how to choose a group activity are important for the group, as they are for any family. When given a choice for Christmas dinner, the residents at one group home choose the traditional turkey dinner with the most traditional of accessories, thereby confirming their identity as a family group. Social workers who look to family rituals for determining how a family operates might well look to how community residents make choices as a group; even more telling is what few choices are left for them to make.

THE METAPHOR OF THE FAMILY: TO HIDE THE NAME OF THE FATHER

It has been shown that the metaphor of the family has been used implicitly and explicitly in defining community residences, and that an understanding of family dynamics can lead to a better understanding of the daily operation of the residence. However, while families are decentered by new arrivals or behavior that ruptures the social scheme designed by the Father (Deleuze and Guattari, 1986, p. 97), community residences are structured by external funding sources which provide the resources and the rules to keep the social control centered in the name of the Father. Use of the metaphor of the family for a community residence allows everyone—the residents, the staff, the social planners, and the families of the clients—to deny the elements of social control that underlie the community residence. From denial of adult sexuality through the use of double bedrooms to the potential for staff to define any deviant behavior as mental illness, the community residence is a powerful strategy for the social control of disabled people. By keeping clients in one place and under surveillance, bureaucrats can minimize interactions between clients and the community. The mentally ill remain hidden, under the eye of the Father, and away from public attention. To the extent that such surveillance is the base of power for those who act in the name of the Father, then it must be questioned as a mastery of the Other (Pfohl and Gordon, 1986). Mastery of the Other is not what social workers believe they do, so they deny their own dominance of others. They block from their awareness their role as agents of the government where this dominance is built into their jobs. All engaged in the control of the disabled must question their own social practice which allows them to objectify the other by naming them as mentally ill and by constructing social spaces in which the desires of the Other are ignored. In humanistic terms we believe ourselves to be individuals burdened by the social constructs around us. Yet a closer examination of one construct—"community residence"—illustrates that our professional practice is so enmeshed with the construct that we can unknowingly be handmaidens to the law of the Father.

While acknowledging the need for some social control of people whose immediate behavior requires control for personal and public safety, social workers must increase public awareness that mental illness does not mean that constant social control is needed. Programs like the clubhouse of New York City's Fountain House, based on rehabilitation model, encourage member control of the social environment and place a demand on those with mental illness to learn and internalize social controls rather than rely on external constraints. The potential for those with mental illness to control their own living spaces and to rely on their own desires for housemates does not fit with the tradition of social control, exclusion, and policy in the name of the Father. If professional practice is to be decentered rather than controlled by the Father, then those engaged in public policy must re-examine their practice, looking beyond metaphors like the family to describe the community residence. To decenter "implies an escape from those philosophical standpoints which have taken consciousness as . . . a given" (Giddens, 1979, p. 47). However constructive understanding the residences as a family may be for daily interventions, the metaphor also locks us into a particular view of the world and protects each of us from viewing our own power and dominance as agents of the Father.

Finally, it has been shown how the simulacra of the family effects the community residence and how the metaphor of family hides elements of social control. I would like to suggest that the metaphor of community residence, with all the ramifications that have been explored here, now be reversed to be used as a lens for exploring the family. Again, in this style of analysis, what is excluded is what is important. If the family is viewed as a community residence then what is most missing is the financial support to maintain the family at an adequate standard of living. Governments appear to grant money where social control, however hidden, is part of the agenda as it is with mentally ill who live in the community residences. But in this country there are no family/child subsidies and no monetary concern for seemingly harmless dependents; perhaps it is because women and children are not targets for social control.

I leave to you the reader the ongoing effort to re-examine the family through different metaphors. The exercise of changing metaphors or lens to explore social practice is necessary for social workers who are engaged daily in the lives of others. Such deconstruction is a way we can assure an awareness of the heterogeneous understandings of the world and can avoid our comfortable routines which hide the privilege and power of our daily practice.

BIBLIOGRAPHY

Alcoff, L. (1989). Cultural Feminism versus post-structuralism. In M. Malson, J. O'Barr, S. Westphal-Wihl, & M. Wyer (Eds.) *Feminist Theory in Practice and Process*. Chicago: University of Chicago Press.

Anderson, H. & Goolishian, H. (1988). Human systems as linguistic systems:

Preliminary and evolving ideas about the implication for clinical theory. Family Process. *27* (4), 371-393.

Barthes, R. (1983). *Mythologies*. New York: Hill & Wang.

Blanch, A., Carling, P., & Ridgway, P. (1988). Normal housing with specialized supports: A psychiatric rehabilitation approach to living in the community. *Rehabilitation Journal*. *33*(1), 47-55.

Deleuze, G. & Guattari, F. (1983). *Anti-Oedipus: Capitalism & schizophrenia*. Minneapolis: University of Minnesota Press.

Efran, J., Lukens, R., & Lukens, M. (1988). Constructivism: What's in it for you. *The Family Therapy Networker*. Sept./Oct. 29-35.

Foucault, M. (1973). *Madness & civilization*. New York: Vintage Books.

Giddens, A. (1984). *The Constitution of society*. Berkeley: University of California Press.

Giddens, A. (1979). *Central problems in social theory*. Berkeley: University of California Press.

Harbin, H. (1988). The family and the psychiatric hospital. In J. Schwartzman (Ed.). *Families and other systems*. New York: Guilford Press.

Harlan, M. (1989). Aristotle's shadow: "models, metaphors, and myths." *The New York Times*. Oct. 22, (E) 24.

Harries, K. (1990). Our analgesic culture [Review of the presence of myth]. *The New York Times Book Review*. Jan. 14, p. 24.

Lakoff, G., & Johnson, M. (1980). *Metaphors we live by*. Chicago: University of Chicago Press.

Pfohl, S. & Gordon, A. (1986). Criminological displacements: toward a sociological deconstruction. *Social Problems*. 33(6), 401-419.

A Three Step Plan
for African-American Families
Involved with Foster Care:
Sibling Therapy, Mothers' Group Therapy,
Family Therapy

Karen Gail Lewis

INTRODUCTION

Over the years, there have been many ideas about the cause of recidivism and how to break the cycle.[1] Unfortunately, the focus most often is on only one piece of the cycle. But the circularity of placement-reunification-placement pattern suggests that to be successful, interventions must be related to the gestalt of the experience. At the very least, this includes the federal to local government, The Agency, mother, and the children.

To do justice to the topic of African-American families and foster care, there needs to be consideration of the broader social and economic issues within the country. There also needs to be consideration of the possible racist underpinnings that may account for the relatively higher rate of foster care for black families. Although these issues are poignant to the whole topic of foster care, this paper will isolate one aspect of recidivism and present a multi-level systemic treatment approach. First there will be a descriptive of the cyclical pattern surrounding the recidivism. Then a three step treatment plan will be described: sibling therapy where the children learn to recognize their role in returning home and to express their feelings in less destructive ways; mothers' group therapy where mothers learn to

Karen Gail Lewis, ACSW, EdD, is in private practice and on the faculty of Johns Hopkins School of Medicine, Department of Child and Adolescent Psychiatry, 1107 Spring Street, Silver Spring, MD 20910.

An earlier version of this paper was presented at the Black Family Summit Conference, Columbia, South Carolina, 1989.

135

feel more competent as a parent and become better connected to their extended family, peer group, and their community; and family therapy where mother and children meet together focusing on issues specifically related to improving the chance of a successful reunification. This three step plan is aimed at families with children under 14 years of age.

THE CYCLICAL PATTERN

A children's protective service (hereafter called The Agency) has the responsibility for removing children from their home when their mother is found to be unable to adequately care for them.[2] She may have abused them or been so involved in her self abuse of illness (e.g., drugs, alcohol, depression, mental illness) that she neglected them. The Agency must then place the children in foster homes, usually in separate homes (Heger, 1988). Often a troubled mother does not receive separate services, e.g., drug treatment, homemaker services, individual therapy. While she may have periodic visitation with her children, if the children are in different foster homes, she may have to see them separately, decreasing the frequency for seeing each child. This also means the children may not get to see each other, for the court seldom mandates that the siblings must visit with each other (Heger, 1988).

The content and quality of the visits are limited by the artificialness of the setting, such as in the social worker's office, a foster home, a park. This presents at least two major glitches. Even if mother gets to visit with all of her children together, their excitement in being with her may lead to their vociferously vying for her attention with escalating friction. Under the best of conditions, a mother tries to be a good parent to each child yet probably feels incompetent to give quality attention to any of the demanding children. The second glitch is that mother's behaviors and responses are bound to be shaped by the awkwardness of having a judgmental spectator. The reality is that the social worker's responsibility is to judge mother's ability to deal with her children.

Even when the visits go smoothly and the children are returned home, the old problems remain: mother's emotional, financial, social, and environmental problems: problems between mother and each child; each child's individual and social problems; as well as problems among the siblings. The children have the additional stress of returning to their former school and re-adjusting to their peers. Not having skills for expressing their feelings of anger, confusion, and sadness verbally, they explode in their most familiar language — fighting and screaming (Minuchin, Montalvo, Guerney, Rosman, & Schumer, 1967). As conflict between the children increases, mother resorts to her former behavior for dealing with stress — alcohol, drugs, withdrawal, etc. That of course, leads back to the beginning of this cycle with the children being placed in a foster home because of mother's abuse or neglect.

CHILDREN'S ROLE IN RECIDIVISM

The children's role in recidivism, specifically as it relates to mother's functioning, has been a neglected subject. This does not intend to blame children for their placement, only to present one aspect that is never discussed. Certainly no social worker would willingly give children the responsibility for such a major decision as to whether they should be returned to their mother, yet in fact, that is what often happens. Some children, so angry at mother that they want to punish her, misbehave, proving mother is not capable of handling them. On the other hand, other children are so solicitous of their mother they are on their very best behavior during visits. Most often, though, there is no conscious intent in the quality of the children's behavior with mother. They may be emotionally pained children whose only expression of their hurt is through their activeness and aggression. Their out of control behavior may reflect how out of control they feel about their whole life. Traditional child psychology is inadequate for explaining their "problems." These children should not be viewed through a middle class lens.

CHILDREN FROM CHAOTIC HOMES

Children from disadvantaged, underorganized (Aponte, 1976), low socioeconomic families tend to be action oriented with no focus to their behavior. They do not expect to be heard and if heard, they do not expect a response. The volume of a voice is more important than the content. They have no negotiating skills so they do not expect resolutions to any conflict. Fighting is a primary means of relating (Minuchin, et al., 1967). Although there is much apparent conflict between these children, the meaning of the fighting is not always so apparent. Since fighting is a primary form of communication, deciphering the communication is crucial. Some of the more common meanings include the following:

- *predictability*. In their chaotic uncertain world, there is safety and familiarity in the predictability of the fights. Siblings know how a fight will begin who will initiate it, how the other will respond, who will do what next, and how it will end.

- *sense of competence*. Regardless of who wins the fight, there is a satisfaction in the initiating. Starting the fight is a way to take charge of something in their life they do not like. "The competence comes not from the winning but from the attack" (Minuchin et al., 1967, p. 294).
- *safe deflection of anger*. In these families, open expression of anger is not safe. Parents are bigger, stronger and can do fatal damage. It is not an equal battle. Deflecting the anger towards a sibling is safer; the retaliation is not so brutal nor so final; they are familiar with the normal sibling alternation between fighting and playing.
- *expression of affect*. In their world, open expression of affect is not valued. Fighting, though, is a socially acceptable means of making contact. Also, since these children externalize their feelings, fighting can diffuse their tension, fear, anger, and hopelessness.
- *avoidance of silence*. Noise and movement are a reassurance of their own presence and that of others. Silence can be seen as abandonment. Further, silence leaves too much room for unacceptable affect to surface.

Fighting, then, is a way to stay connected or bonded (Bank & Kahn, 1982; Lewis, 1986a). Siblings are emotionally engaged as long as they hit and shout, which reinforce their presence in each other's life. At some point, though, the fighting can move beyond a form of connection and become cruel, abusive, or incestuous.

To the other extreme are the children from chaotic homes who have not developed a bonding; they pull away from each other. While there is no fighting, there is also no sense of relatedness; their isolation is intended as a self-protection. They have no recognition that they share the same pain; they can not imagine they have anything to learn from each other. In fact, in some disengaged families, with multiple comings and goings, the siblings may not even know each other's names or ages.

STEP ONE: SIBLING THERAPY

Sibling therapy is a forum for bringing brothers and sisters together in the same room to deal with mutual problems. A relatively new concept, sibling therapy has been used with children and adults with a wide range of problems (Kahn & Lewis, 1988).

The goals of sibling therapy with African-American children hoping to be returned to their family unit need to be circumscribed. It is possible that each child has multiple problems — intrapsychic, interpersonal, social, academic, economic, etc. That, together with mother's problems, extended family problems, current family adjustment, prior family crises, overt and covert racism, leave the children burdened beyond any reasonable comprehension. With such global problems, therapy can feel futile. Add to that, the fact that underorganized families typically do not remain in therapy for any length of time (Aponte & Van Deusen, 1981). The social worker may feel overwhelmed, same as the children; therapy may seem a mission impossible.

In this type of sibling therapy, it is important to focus primarily on the issues that will help the family most immediately, choosing problems that need immediate attention and that have a chance for immediate results. With children in foster care, a primary question is, What are the basic steps, relating only to the children, that are necessary to make a smooth transition back to their home? At the least, areas to be targeted for therapy should include working with the schools to help the children academically and socially; improving the daily interactions among the siblings; and emphasizing mutuality—what affects one will affect them all.

The social worker needs to contact both the new and old schools in preparation for the children's transfer. The teachers need to be alerted to possible problems with social adjustment in the new setting and with differences in class content. When at all possible, taking the children to visit the new school before the placement is a useful way to help the transition go more smoothly. During the sibling therapy, it is helpful to encourage the children to talk to each other about their changed school, new classmates, and the class work. The sharing and mutual problem solving serve to strengthen their concern for each other.

For helping the children improve their daily interactions and emphasizing their mutuality, there are specific issues that need to be addressed:

a. an understanding of why they were removed from their mother
b. their feelings about the breakup of their home
c. their guilt for causing the breakup—sorting out how much was their fault and how much was not
d. their blame of each other for the breakup
e. their separation from each other
f. their adjustment to the new home, neighborhood, school
g. a discussion of the visitations—what went well and what they believe needs to be changed
h. their feelings about returning home and what changes they can make to help the family run smoother if they do return
i. things they like about each other

    j. their learning to play and talk together
    k. their learning to translate feelings into words so they can say what
       they really mean or ask directly for what they need and want.

There are many other important issues, but they can wait. For instance, intrapsychic problems take a very long time to solve and often are not even reachable until daily life settles down.

This list seems long and very complicated for young children, yet it is not impossible to make inroads in all of the above within a few months. Clearly, none of the topics can be dealt with completely, but they each can be continuously raised and the interrelationship between the issues underscored. Even just a cognitive understanding gives children some sense of participation, if not control, over their otherwise powerless position in the family. Above age three or four, children can see the direct connection that if two of them fight, mother might walk out, or if one child feels lonely, perhaps another is feeling the same thing. They may not be able to make changes in their behavior, but seeing the connection between the issues and the advantage of their working together as a unit will make them more readily available to learn how to make the changes. At the same time, they need to understand that they are only one part of the family. Regardless what they do, mother may not be able to do her part. When that happens, they need much reassurance that if they do not return home, it is not their fault.

Therapy can become a safe forum for their expression of rage and helplessness; they can learn alternative ways of dealing with their feelings rather than hurting each other. As they begin to verbally share their feelings, they learn that they are not alone. Breaking the emotional isolation is also an important step in changing the behavior. While the type of interactions between the children may not change dramatically, the quality can. For example, the children may move from nasty fighting with the intent of venting their anger onto each other to play-fighting as a way of sharing their mutual anger.

Sibling therapy, while using some cognitive teaching and discussion, relies heavily on activity and play therapy. Descriptions of the actual therapy interventions have been presented elsewhere (Lewis, 1986a; 1986c), as well as the role of the therapist (Lewis, 1986b). Briefly, the leader must be active, expecting noise and a high activity level in the room. The leader must take a directive role, focusing the play and the discussion to the poignant topics, such as asking, "I know your mother didn't show up for her promised visit last week; do you think maybe you were angry at her and that is why you burned your sister's dress?" The children do not need just a reflection of their feelings: they need direct confrontation with the vital issues in their life. For children too young for such a conversation, the same idea can be played out with dolls; the therapist enacts a scene with the dolls that demonstrates the two related ideas. Young children will let you know through their comments or participation in the play if your comments are accurate. If so, then the next play scene can follow up on the feelings of the disappointed child. There are also some techniques for helping silent and "resistant" children (Lewis, 1986c).

BLACK MOTHERS

Poor, African-American, under-educated, single, women from urban cities make up a disproportionate percentage of mothers whose children are placed in foster homes (Gurak, Smith, & Goldson, 1982; Jenkins & Norman, 1972; Shyne & Schroeder, 1978). Yet,

> Children do not come into care because their parents are poor or black or sick. . . . .poverty is a necessary but not a sufficient condition for placement. It is the marginal family, whose characteristics and social circumstances are such that it cannot sustain further stress, which utilizes the placement system as a last resort when its own fragile supports break down. (Jenkins & Norman, 1972, p. 19)

Any parent with emotionally stressed or disturbed children will have difficulty with them. Mothers with their own problems will have less skills in dealing with their troubled children. Add to this the fact that mother often is un(under)employed, untrained, and faced with the effects of a four-fold prejudice: being black, being female, being a single parent, being poor. In addition, too often she is emotionally cut off from her family and social community. Feeling overwhelmed and incompetent to deal with all of the problems, she may choose her familiar escape route (drugs, etc.).

The social worker needs to have an understanding of black families. While there is diversity among black families (not all blacks are alike), there are many cultural similarities (Hines & Boyd-Franklin, 1982). Relevant to the topic here, most blacks share an African legacy which values survival of the tribe over the individual (Boyd-Franklin, 1989); they endured institutional racism and discrimination; they are part of a "victim system" (Pinderhughes, 1982). Yet, there are many strengths: flexible family roles; value of education and achievement, despite social constraints that deter from these values; strong spiritual and religious beliefs; and a strong kinship bond and loyalty to family, related or not (Boyd-Franklin, 1989; McAdoo, 1980). Traditionally, blacks survival has been attributed to the strength of their kinship bonds (Boyd-Franklin, 1989;

McAdoo & McAdoo, 1985). The extended family can be important in maintaining economic as well as emotional stability. The extended family often includes non-blood related members since blacks historically have had their own informal adoptions, taking in each other's children when needed (Boyd-Franklin, 1989). The concept of foster care, losing one's child to an unknown family, cuts across the very core of black family interdependence, for a child to go in a foster home—a stranger's family—suggests the mother's fragile supports have broken down, have gone beyond a tolerable stress level.

Throughout the centuries, black women have been identified with mothering and caretaking (McCray, 1980; Staples, 1973). Losing her children may be the ultimate sign of having lost total control over her life. When that happens, she needs help in becoming empowered as a person and as a woman; she needs help in regaining her family ties and in resuming her role as a nurturing mother to her children. One potent way to help women do this is through the medium of group therapy.

STEP TWO: MOTHERS' GROUP THERAPY

The medium of group therapy is consistent with the traditional African-American world view that puts the group before its members; "I am because we are; and because we are, therefore, I am" (Mbiti, 1969, p. 108). Group therapy can offer a syntonic means of helping mothers whose children have been removed to a foster home.

The mothers' group therapy runs concurrent with the sibling therapy. Four to eight women meet for eight to twelve weeks with others experiencing the same feelings of shame, helplessness, and anger. For some women, this is the first time they have talked with others about losing their children. The camaraderie that develops becomes a chink in their isolation. The group provides such emotional and social supports that often the women continue to meet informally after the therapy is over.

During the first session, the social worker, taking a directive role, (re)explains to each woman the reasons for the removal of her children and what changes must occur before they can be returned. This lets the other women know they are all there for similar reasons and becomes a kick off point for each to tell her story. The affect during this period is usually one of accusatory anger at The Agency and of the women's helplessness in the face of white bureaucracy. The social worker must not be defensive; correcting the "facts" can occur later. At this stage, the goal is for the women to feel heard by the social worker and by each other. The sharing becomes a basis for developing a unifying bond.

By the third or fourth session, the social worker can begin directing the discussion to specific topics related to the steps the women need to take to get their children back. This may include mutual problem solving around personal problems, relationships, living arrangements, employment, etc. Issues that arise during visitations or questions on how to relate or discipline better can be discussed in the group.

Once the women are past their initial hostility at having to be in the group, several important questions should be raised. Whose idea was the placement? Do the mothers see The Agency as helping their child or as usurping their parental rights? This discussion may free some mothers to express their relief from the pressure of dealing with their children while their own lives are so chaotic. Others, though, may feel the placement as a personal violation. Discussions should also include topics such as their competency as mothers, as women, as African-American. Certainly issues of drug or alcohol dependency will arise as they begin to trust each other. There is as a better chance for success if the group suggests and supports one or several women seek help than if a social worker mandates it.* Another crucial topic is the women recognizing themes for women; many women turn their anger inward, becoming depressed or suicidal or numb it through an addiction. Reading parts of *A Dance of Anger* (Lerner, 1985) together during the group can be bonding and affirming while decreasing the embarrassment of those who have difficulty with reading.

Since the primary intent of the separation is to help the mothers become more conscientious parents, they can begin working on this even though their children are not living with them. In fact, it may be easier for the mothers since they do not have the daily pressure of dealing with all of the children at once.

There are three major areas where they can begin practicing being more competent parents: dealing with the foster parents; dealing with the schools; and rebuilding contact with their extended family, church, and community.

Foster Parents

An open channel between mother and the foster parents augers well for a smooth transition into and back out of the foster home. Losing one's children is bound to make any parent feel defensive and inadequate. Letting mother have contact with the foster mother gives her a continuing role so she does not feel totally ineffectual. However, she may be so angry about the removal of her children or so out of control that the children's whereabouts must remain secret. Still, there are ways to help her show

---

*Editor's Note: See Walker and Small in this issue.

interest in and practice being more involved with her children, e.g., supervised telephone calls, or letters via the social worker—both of which protect the foster family's privacy. Mother can be helped to inquire about her children and to share information about them with the foster family, such as sharing their favorite foods or sleeping habits. While the two mothers may be mutually hostile, they need to understand that they must work together to help the children.

The foster parents need to understand the importance of mother's involvement, however, peripheral, yet they may also need protection from mother. This can be done by assuring that all contact will occur only through the social worker and at pre-scheduled times. Further, they can be coached that they need only to listen to mother's input; they do not have to contradict mother or argue with her.

Schools

Many mothers avoid contact with teachers because of the residual fear from their own schools days; they may feel inadequate in talking with teachers. Yet, it is important for the mothers to show more interest in their children's school. The women can be reminded of the high value black families have always placed on education; they need to be reminded that education is necessary to get ahead in life; they probably do not need to be reminded that they all want their children to get further ahead in life than they have.

The social worker can help the mothers prepare questions to ask the teacher. The mothers can practice with each other what they would say to a teacher and role play various ways to approach a teacher. If there is a concern about a mother being inappropriate with a teacher, the same protective measures as used with the foster family can be used with the teacher, e.g., pre-arranged supervised telephone conversations or letters.

Family, Church, and Community

Since the extended family is very important in African-American families, the social worker needs to ask who else is involved in the woman's life. Are her parents alive? Does she have any siblings? Is she close with her sister-in-law or her cousins? The inquiry should include friends and religious community which often is a stabilizing force for black families. The larger the network the social worker can identify, the larger the pool of support from which to cull help. These people can be invited into later family sessions or individual sessions with the mother (Haber, 1978). The goals for the collaborative sessions should be to mobilize the support system to help mother in concrete or emotional ways. If a mother has dropped out of a religious group, she should be encouraged to visit a church with one of the other group members or the group can attend together.

Group therapy can become a place for the women to feel heard, to try new behaviors, to learn interpersonal social skills. As the women learn that others value what they have to offer, they develop a sense of worthiness and competence. Feeling better about themselves as women is an important step in helping them work towards feeling better about themselves as mothers.

STEP THREE: BEGINNING THE REUNIFICATION THROUGH FAMILY THERAPY

As the children and mother make progress in their respective therapies, while still living apart, they meet together weekly for family therapy. The goals for mother should include learning how to play and have fun with her children and how to discipline appropriately. The goals for the children should include being able to talk more easily about their feelings and to ask for what they want from each other without fighting or screaming.

The social worker, being directive, uses discussions and play to deal with specific problems that interfere with the family's chance for reunification. They can role play family situations with mother and children sometimes switching roles as they experiment with creating different responses to typical scenes. This is an especially fun exercise for children and can be very effective in stretching each person's options for new behaviors.

When the children misbehave during a therapy session, the mother needs to be the one to reprimand them. The social worker may offer phrases for the mother to say or suggest an action she could take, but mother must be the one to directly respond to the children. If the children do not listen, the social worker can reinforce mother's message, e.g., "Lotti, your mother told you not to do that." However, it is important that the social worker not take over mother's role.

If the family therapy is going well, the children may be returned to mother, but the treatment should continue for some time beyond the reunification.

CONCLUSIONS

This paper proposes a three step approach to reunification of the family after foster placement. This preventive approach can be used with all families but may be especially useful with first time placements. The basic premise is that if the children are less agitated by their melange of feelings, they will be more manageable when they return home; mother, then, will feel less overwhelmed and perhaps be better able to take control of the family. A corollary is that reunification will be smoother if (1) mother feels heard and valued and if she begins to develop an appropriate social network; (2) if the children are less disturbed, less angry at mother, and less angry at each other; (3) if the children behave better so mother has a less difficult time controlling them; (4) if the home life includes some playful moments between mother and her children.

Some children, though, may never be returned to their mother. For those who have no bonding or only a tenuous bond with their siblings, building or strengthening this connection can be crucial for their future adjustment. If their mothers are not able to learn how to provide them with the nurturance they need and deserve, they can learn to provide a sense of family for each other. If a strong sibling connection can be created or reinforced, they will have an on-going, consistent support system. As they encounter difficult years ahead, which may include a long road of multiple separations and placements, they will have the benefit of knowing that some family member is beside them. This can be especially important if they never return to their mother. Whether they end up living together or in separate foster homes, they will have this on-going sense of familyness and connectedness. Knowing that a brother or sister cares about them may take the edge off the loneliness and isolation resulting from parental deprivation.

NOTES

1. It is interesting to note that the major journals dealing with foster care have few articles written after the 1960's dealing specifically with the recidivism rate and with African-American children—this despite the fact that more than half of the children in foster care are black (Eastman, 1985).

2. The term mother is used because of the preponderance of single mother-headed families. However, many of the issues are the same when mother and father live together.

REFERENCES

Aponte, H. (1976). Underorganization in the poor family. In P. Guerin (Ed.) *Family therapy: Theory and practice.* New York: Gardner.

Aponte, H. & Van Deusen, J. (1981). Structural family therapy. In A. Gurman & D. Kniskern (Eds.), *Handbook of family therapy.* New York: Brunner/Mazel.

Bank, S. & Kahn, M. (1982). *The sibling bond.* New York: Basic Books.

Boyd-Franklin, N. (1989). *Black families in therapy.* New York: Guilford.

Eastman, K.S. (9185). Foster families: A comprehensive bibliography. *Child welfare, 64*, 6, 565-585.

Gurak, D.T., Smith, D.A., & Goldson, M.F. (1982). *The minority foster child: A comparative study of Hispanic, black and white children*. New York: Hispanic Research Center Fordham University.

Haber, R. (1987). Friends in family therapy: Use of a neglected resource. *Family Process, 26*, 269-281.

Hegar, R. (1988). Legal and social work approaches to sibling separation in foster care. *Child Welfare, 67*, 2, 113-121.

Hines, P.M. & Boyd-Franklin, N. (1982). Black families. In M. McGoldrick, J. Pearce, & J. Giordano (Eds.), *Ethnicity and family therapy*. New York: Guilford.

Jenkins, S. & Norman, E. (1972). *Filial deprivation and foster care*. New York: Columbia Press.

Kahn, M. & Lewis, K.G. (Eds.) (1988). *Siblings in therapy: Life span and clinical issues*. New York: Norton.

Lerner, H.G. (1985). *The dance of anger*. New York: Harper & Row.

Lewis, K.G. (1986a). Sibling therapy with multiproblem families. *Journal of Marital and Family Therapy, 12*, 3, 291-300.

Lewis, K.G. (1986b). Sibling therapy with children in foster homes. In L. Combrinck-Graham (Ed.), *Treating young children in family therapy*. Rockville, MD.: Aspen.

Lewis, K.G. (1986c). Systemic play therapy: A tool for social work consultation to inner-city community mental health centers. *Journal of Independent Social Work, 1*, 2, 33-43.

Mbiti, J.S. (1969). *African religions and philosophies*. Garden City, NY: Anchor Books.

McAdoo, H.P. (1980). Black mothers and the extended family support network. In La Frances Rodgers-Rose (Ed.), *The black woman*. Beverly Hills: Sage.

McAdoo, H.P. & McAdoo, J.L. (Eds.) (1985). *Black children: Social educational and parental environments*. Beverly Hills: Sage.

McCray, C.A. (1980). The black woman and family roles. In La Frances Rodgers-Rose (Ed.), *The black woman*. Beverly Hills: Sage.

Minuchin, S., Montalvo, B., Guerney, B.G., Jr., Rosman, B.L., & Schumer, F. (1967). *Families of the slums: An exploration of their structure and treatment*. New York: Basic Books.

Pinderhughes, E. (1982). Afro-American families and the victim system. In M. McGoldrick, J.K. Pearce, & J. Giordano (Eds.) *Ethnicity and family therapy*. New York: Guilford.

Shyne, A.W. & Schroeder, A.G. (1978). *National study of social services to children and their families: Overview*. Washington, D.C.: U.S. Government Printing Office.

Staples, R. (1973). *The black woman in American: Sex, marriage, and the family*. Chicago: Nelson Hall.

Every Clinical Social Worker Is in Post-Adoption Practice

Ann Hartman

The field of adoption has long been considered a special area within child welfare. Social workers in other fields of practice and clinical social workers in agencies or independent practice have tended to consign expertise about adoption to child welfare practitioners or adoption specialists and to consider issues around adoption as irrelevant to their practice.

The fact is, however, that everyone in practice, certainly everyone offering counseling or clinical services under any auspice is faced daily with adoption issues. A substantial portion of our clients are adoptees or are sons, daughters, birth parents, adoptive parents, spouses, siblings of or are otherwise closely related to an adoptee. To gain a sense of the extent to which adoption touches every clinician's practice, it is only necessary to remember that there are between two and three million adoptees in this country! and then to multiply that by the number of people closely connected to those millions

Until fairly recently, clinicians have often failed to recognize adoption when it is a part of an individual's or family's life. Further, even when the adoption is identified, its significance has frequently been ignored. H.D. Kirk (1964) in his pioneering study of adoption and adoptive families discovered that those who understood and accepted the difference between adoption and biological parenting tended to be the most successful adoptive parents.

Such parents, however, were taking a position quite different from the discourse and the mythology upon which much of adoption practice was based. The goal of traditional adoption practice was to make adoption as much as possible like biological parenting. In the process, the differences between the two tended to be denied. This model of adoption was apparent in the effort to match a child physically to the parents, to cut off and

Ann Hartman is Dean, School of Social Work, Smith College, Northhampton, MA 01060.

make insignificant the child's biological roots and preadoption experience, and to get the agency out of the family's life as quickly as possible. Post-adoption services to families were minimal and brief on the assumption that because adoptive families were just like any other family, they didn't need any special help.

Most adoptive families, many of whom have suffered greatly over their infertility and the loss of their dream for a biological child, were glad to join the adoption agencies in denying the difference between adopting and giving birth. This discourse was powerful and also reassuring as it avoided and denied the complexities, the pain, the losses that are also a part of adoption. It is certainly understandable that the general public and mental health professionals joined with the families and the adoption experts and accepted the myth that adoption was not *really* different. It may be, however, that as with the adoptive families in Kirk's study, the more understanding and accepting therapists are of the reality that adoption is different the more successful they have been in working with individuals and families who have an important connection with adoption.

The growing adoptees' rights movement and the voices of adoptees telling their stories have changed and challenged the adoption myths. Adoptees and birth parents are teaching mental health practitioners about adoption. Clinical theory emanating from the family therapy movement about the importance of family connections and the reverberations of unresolved loss and the destructiveness of secrets in the lives of individuals and families gave support to the experiences reported by adoptees. The attention of clinicians and researchers has thus been drawn to the importance of adoption through the media's reporting on the lives of adopted people; books and articles have also contributed to our understanding of and ability to help around adoption issues (Brodzinsky and Schechter, 1990; Sorosky, Baran, and Pannor, 1984).

In this paper, two major themes—loss and identity—that emerge around adoption, will be explored. Implications for family centered practice and interventive strategies will be discussed and illustrated through case examples drawn from general family centered practice.

As these themes are pursued and the clients who have important connections with adoption are introduced, it is hoped that it will become evident that everyone in direct practice with individuals and families is in post-adoption practice. Focus will be primarily on infant adoption and its impact on adoptees, birth parents, and those close to them. The special issues in working with adoptive families in conjoint family therapy have been explored elsewhere (Hartman and Laird, 1990).

THE THEME OF LOSS

The central theme in adoption is loss. Everyone in the adoption triangle, the adoptee, the birth parents, and the adoptive parents have experienced a major loss. The adoptees have lost their biological family, the birth parents have lost their child, and the adoptive parents have lost the biological children they had anticipated they would have. The members of the adoption triangle and those who are close to them are affected by this universal experience of loss.

Perhaps even more significant than the losses is the fact that for the adoptee, birth parent, and adoptive parents, their losses have not been recognized or validated. For many the loss is quiet, secret, unshared and unresolved. Frequently, the loss has been handled by denial and repression. Denial around adoption has been in part iatrogenic, as adoptees, birth parents, and adoptive parents have been involved with a system of adoption based on denial and have worked with professionals who encouraged and reinforced the denial, failing to recognize the very real pain and loss. Adoptees' wish to search has been invalidated as agency workers, carefully guarding records, have interpreted that wish as problematic or even a symptom of disturbance and a poor adoption. The gravity and extent of the loss and mourning suffered by a birth parent in relinquishing a child has been invalidated by social workers who have falsely reassured them saying, "You'll forget, put this behind you and go on with your life."

Adoptive parents have worked with adoption workers who are so invested in the successful and joyful placement of a baby that they do not want to know about the sometimes abiding sense of disappointment, about the bitter sweet joy of adoption that may also reawaken the longing for the biological child. Clinicians, because of their own denial, may have little or no awareness of the importance of this in their clients' lives or of the relevance of the adoption to the presenting problems. If the clinician fails to discover the presence of the adoption issue or joins that client's denial, it may well be that the core issue in the person's life is bypassed.

Adoptees and Loss

Claire sought help almost three years after the sudden death of her husband. A successful professional woman in her early 40s, she was severely depressed and had been unable to move beyond the loss. She was embarrassed and apologetic about seeking help. She thought she ought to be feeling better but if anything, she was worse.

The first three sessions focused on her husband, the marriage, and her grieving. She seemed totally caught in the mourning process. In the fourth session, the therapist realized, much to her surprise, that she had failed to get any family history. This was very different from her general way of working and she recognized that something about the client had "warned her off" her usual path. She proceeded to ask about Claire's family and learned, after some discussion, that the client was adopted. Could it be that the inability to even begin to resolve the loss of her husband was related to that earlier loss, the loss of her birth parents? The client was very disinterested in talking about her origins, maintaining that it was entirely irrelevant to her current grief and her situation. At this point, it would have been easy to accept her position that the adoption was without consequence.

The worker, however, persisted and over the next months, the story began to unfold. Claire really knew little about her beginnings except that her's was a private adoption through a cousin of her father. She supposed her birth mother was unmarried but was not sure. She thought she was about 18 months old when she was adopted and did not know where she had spent the first year and a half of her life. She was always described by her family as "sober sides" and she had seen many pictures in family albums of a grave, unsmiling toddler and child. Although Claire continued to feel this was all beside the point, the worker continued to turn the focus to her origins and finally, Claire did begin to allow herself to become more curious about her past. The turning point came when, quite unexpectedly, she decided to call the cousin who had told her adoptive parents about her. Thus she began to fashion a new and more complete adoption story.

She learned that her birth mother had been a good friend of the cousin. She discovered that her mother, a self-supporting working woman in her early 30s, had tried to keep her. This was long before this was an acceptable thing to do. Her mother had continued to work but kept her daughter with her in her small apartment and arranged for sitters. She had little support, except from Claire's future adoptive parents' cousin and another friend. Finally, after eighteen months, she arranged the private adoption through her friend who knew that Claire's adoptive parents were seeking a child. The fact that her birth mother had tried to keep her, against all odds, had great meaning to her. Claire began to get in touch with the loss she experienced as a toddler and to realize how depressed she was as a young child.

Interestingly enough, these explorations made her feel closer to her adoptive parents. For the first time she talked about the adoption with her mother and father and arranged to spend her vacation with them, something she had not done in many years. Her depression slowly abated as the original loss was discovered, explored, and validated. She began to consider searching for her birth mother.

The importance of the adoption story in a person's life is well illustrated in this case. Both individual and family therapists are turning their attention to narratives and stories of how people construct their lives and to the process of therapy as a construction of a new story (Laird, 1989). Through the storying and restorying process, in and out of therapy, people make and remake the meaning of their lives (Carlsen, 1988). When Claire came to therapy, her adoption was largely unstoried and full of gaps. It carried a strong implication of rejection by her mother. She had never, within memory, talked about the adoption with her parents. The lack of information about where she had spent the first 18 months of her life exaggerated her sense of discontinuity. She was ashamed of being called "sober sides" feeling it reflected her adoptive parents' disappointment in her. This shame was not unlike the shame she now felt about not being able to deal better with her husband's death. Although connections continued to be made to her current situation, the most powerful part of her work was slowly developing a new adoption story which, in turn, gave her a very different view of herself; she constructed a new meaning, not only of her adoption but of her life.

The loss of her birth mother and the implications for this woman's life can be understood from several theoretical perspectives. From a Bowen Family Systems perspective, this loss can be understood as a major cut off. The concept of the "cut off," an emotional break from the family is key in Bowen's theory and is clearly exemplified by a closed adoption being the ultimate cut off. Bowen (1978) suggests that the more complete the cut off, the more intense is the involvement with the absent figures. This is particularly seen in the frequency with which a person who is cut off from significant figures repeats the patterns from beyond the cut off (Bowen, 1976 p. 536). The therapeutic method developed by Bowen and his colleagues of coaching a person to reconnect with important members of their family of origin helps us understand the power and the healing potential of the adoptee search process.

It may also be considered that for this client, the loss of her birth mother and her adoption was in Daniel Stern's (1985) terms, the narrative point of origin, "the potent life-experience that provides the key therapeutic metaphor for understanding and changing the patient's life"(p. 257).

The primary task in therapy according to Stern is to find the narrative point and to reconstruct the narrative. Although Claire was a mature, well functioning woman, there was always about her the deep sense of being a lost child seeking a home. She had found a home with her husband in a fairly late marriage. His death powerfully revived the central metaphor of her life and its associated affects.

Some of these same themes are illustrated in the situation of Sharon, a fifteen-year old who was brought for help by her parents because she was acting out sexually. The family began the first session by reporting that their daughter was adopted but they were sure that had nothing to do with her problem. The major portion of the work with this family was around the construction of the adoption story. The family had told Sharon she was adopted and felt that they had been very open to the discussion. They were amazed to discover how vague she was about her origins and how little she remembered of what they had told her. Work with Sharon and her family included a detailed recounting of every step of the adoption story including the parents' discovery that they were infertile, their decision to adopt, their search for a baby, their trip to an adoption agency in another state where Sharon was adopted, and every detail about the first days with their new daughter. They brought photograph albums which included pictures of every part of the event. They also shared everything they knew about Sharon's parents and, most importantly to Sharon, the fact that her mother, even with the agency's disapproval, took care of her infant daughter the first few days of her life. Sharon said with such feeling, "You mean she held me, she really knew me?" The family planned to take a trip to the agency and talk to the adoption worker who was still on the staff not only to fill in more details about the birth parents but to connect with someone connected with the birth mother.

The importance of the adoption story is demonstrated by the popularity of the book *The Chosen Baby* (Wassen, 1939) written for adoptive parents to read to their children. Of course this fictional story is not the child's own story and was used to supply a story in the vacuum created by the secrecy or lack of information about the adoptee's origins.

As family centered practitioners know, toxic issues may be transmitted down through the generations and thus an adoption in one generation may well reverberate for many years. Of particular significance to a person adopted in infancy is the birth of the first child. At that moment, an adoptee looks for the first time in conscious memory upon the face of a biologically related person. Further, particularly for a female, the birth of a child recreates the mother/child relationship, the relationship severed by their relinquishment. The intense and generally repressed feelings about the birth mother tend to be evoked around the birth of a child and that child may be identified with the lost mother. The adoption thus resonates in the relationship with the first born.

In one situation, Carol, a young woman in a group studying their families of origin, said she was the only child in a large family who had been abused by her mother. In studying her family of origin, it came to light that her mother had been adopted in infancy. In adulthood, Carol had changed her last name out of rebellion and a sense of alienation from her parents. Some rather extensive detective work recalled the fact that she had unconsciously chosen the English translation of her birth grandmother's name. She later revealed that as a child she had come across her mother's adoption papers.

In yet another situation, Janet, another first born daughter in a large family, sought help around relationship problems, identity issues, and low self-esteem. Family of origin work first focused on her complex relationship with her father who had died when she was twenty.

As attention turned to her relationship with her mother, it became evident that there was considerable distance between them and that her mother felt very ambivalent toward this daughter. She was apparently much closer to and more comfortable with the other children. Janet felt that she was somehow different than her siblings. She felt almost an outsider. Her mother had been adopted as an infant but this was never discussed in the family. In time, Janet was able to talk with her mother about the adoption and the two of them began to work together on getting more information about the mother's origins. Although they had a difficult search ahead of them because of the passage of time, the discussion and the attention to the mother's birth as a real person began to diminish Janet's mother's unconscious and very powerful identification of Janet with her birth mother.

The Birth Parent and Loss

We are only beginning to look squarely at the experience of the birth parent who relinquishes a child for adoption. We are beginning to allow ourselves to know that the loss of the child has a lingering impact in the parent's life. It is not something we professionals should have had to learn. We know that the loss of a child, under any circumstance, is one of the most painful to bear. How is it that professionals could have minimized this loss? Was it simply wishful thinking? Was it a hidden feeling that anyone who could give up a baby couldn't really have strong feelings for the child? Or could it be that it was such a painful thing to contemplate that professionals denied the birth parents' pain to protect themselves from pain? In any event, the standard and accepted message to birth parents upon relinquishment as "You must put this behind you and go on with your life."

Recent studies of birth parents, although skewed because of the difficulty of finding unbiased samples, constantly report that many of the birth mothers[2] experience profound and protracted grief and an enduring preoccupation with and concern about the welfare of the child (Deykin, Campbell, Patti, 1984; Winkler and van Keppel, 1984). It is also significant that poor outcomes for the birth mothers were found to be associated in part with the lack of opportunity to express their feelings about the loss. Further, it is important for clinical practitioners who are likely to have among their clients one of the million women who have relinquished a child, to know that 50 percent of the birth mothers in the most intensive study to date reported an increasing sense of loss which extended for as long as thirty years (Winkler and van Keppel, 1984).

Unfortunately, birth mothers who have been reassured by professionals at the time of relinquishment that they will forget have this message reinforced by therapists who fail to recognize the importance of the abiding and unresolved grief and loss. For example, one woman sought help with a variety of problems, including a fifteen year history of alcohol abuse. A genogram quickly revealed the fact that her drinking had begun shortly after she had relinquished a child for adoption. She had been in therapy with three different therapists over the years and none of them had identified the loss of the child as relevant or significant.

In another situation, Beverly, a very troubled young woman living a very chaotic life, sought help stating that she had relinquished a daughter for adoption fourteen years previously. Her reason for seeking help at this time was that her daughter was getting old enough to search for her. Beverly wanted to get herself and her life together just in case her daughter found her. Although the ensuing work with the client was sensitive and skilled, discussion about the lost child and the client's feelings about her were not a part of the therapy.

The experience of the birth mother is the relinquishment of a child must be distinguished from that of parents who lose a child through death. The finality, as painful as it is, facilitates the eventual resolution of the death. The fact that the parent will never see and hold the child again slowly becomes real in the letting-go process. With adoption, the child is lost but not dead; for many, the grief work cannot proceed because the child is somewhere out there and the fantasy of seeing the child again and even of reuniting with the child cannot be relinquished. The experience is perhaps analogous to that of the families of the MIA soldiers in Vietnam whose agony was prolonged for years by the hope that somewhere their loved one is alive.

Birth parents report seeing children on the street or in a store who are the same age and sex as their lost child and wondering, if the child could be theirs. On some level, some search forever. The rather surprising finding that the feelings of loss for many birth mothers become more intense as time goes on may in part be due to the fact that as the child gets older and moves into adolescence and young adulthood, the possibility of a reunion becomes somewhat less remote.

It is very possible to be helpful to birth parents whose post-adoption adjustment has been negatively affected by the loss of a child. First, it is essential to discover the fact that a client once relinquished a child. Family therapists who regularly do genograms in their work are likely to learn about the lost child. The likelihood of learning about the child will be increased when people are listing their children to ask "Were there any other pregnancies?" Few clients come requesting help with this issue and many do not recognize or at least would be unwilling to admit the fact that the relinquishment continues to be a painful and unresolved issue.

Secondly, it can be very helpful when the birth parent finally has an opportunity to talk about the whole experience, to grieve, to cry, to have her feelings accepted and validated. The work of family therapist, Norman Paul, on operational mourning is very helpful in this regard (Paul & Grasser, 1965). Paul believes that many of the people seen by mental health professionals who have difficulty relating to others or who are chronically depressed are suffering from unresolved grief, often unknown to them. In the operational mourning process, the original loss is surfaced through reminiscence, association, or through the use of triggering experiences, and the client is given the opportunity to go through the loss again, this time in a supportive relationship with someone who encourages and accepts the grieving process. Leading the client back to and through the loss is painful for the professional as it seems like "making the client cry." The tears, however, have been stored for years. The birth mother is also helped as she shares her fantasies about the child, her dreams of reunification, her fears about the welfare of the child. Often, the birth mother has been enormously self-critical because of her inability to "forget and go on with her life." She tends to feel there is something wrong with her that she could not do it the "right" way. The acceptance and normalization of these feelings is very relieving and helpful. The operational mourning process takes time, and it is important not to consider the work done after one grieving session.

Thirdly, the issue of reunification should be realistically discussed rather than simply nurtured in fantasy. As was discussed in one study of birth mothers, the need to actually search for the child was most powerful in those who felt forced to relinquish through external pressures. The sense of powerlessness, of not having been in charge, and the helpless anger about this appears to be another important aspect of the response to the loss of the child. A realistic discussion of the possibility and desirability of a search, and encouraging the client to make a decision about what she actually wants to do is very empowering. There is one step a birth mother can take on her own behalf in this situation where her rights to set aside the confidentiality around the adoption are even less than those of the adoptee. She can register herself in the computerized system that has been developed by adoptee search organizations through which adoptees and birth parents may locate each other. This proactive step assures the birth parent that should her child want to find her, she would then be able to do so. She can also return to the agency, if this were an agency adoption, to see if the agency had any more non-identifying information on the child and family that they could share.

Finally, and even more empowering, the client can be encouraged to join Concerned United Birth Parents (CUB) or another self-help organization concerned with adoptive issues. In CUB, the client will be able to join with others who have also relinquished children. She will be able to share her experience and listen to the experiences of others. She can finally talk about this important part of her life that has often been defined as a shameful secret. Joining CUB is also empowering because CUB has been an important force in working for adoption reform, in advocating for the rights of birth parents, and in educating professionals about the issues and conflicts in relinquishing a child. For some birth parents, joining with these publicly articulate and active birth parents can be enormously helpful for someone who has lived with silence, shame, and resignation. Other self-help groups include all the members of the adoption triangle and give birth mothers, even if they can not meet their own child, an opportunity to talk to other adoptees and to learn about their experiences, thoughts and feelings.

ADOPTION AND IDENTITY

A second major theme in adoption, particularly for the adoptee, is the issue of identity. "Who am I?" is an issue for all people as they mature, establish a solid sense of self, as they go through various changes and transitions in their life cycle, as they come to terms with their particular life. The adoptee's effort to answer that question, to establish a firm identity is complicated when there is a cut off from the biological family. As one adoptee poignantly said, "I didn't know what I looked like until I saw my birth mother. It was as if I had to look into a face that looked like my face in order to be able to see my face." Schechter and Bertocci (1990) have referred to the adoptees' "missing experience of likeness-to-self" (p. 88-89) which this adoptee may be expressing. Another adoptee dramatically demonstrated the feeling of emptiness, of the unknown, when her turn came to present her family to a family of origin group. She went to the empty blackboard where in previous meetings group members had drawn their genograms and, pointing to it said, "There's my genogram." She later drew her adoptive family's genogram demonstrating, as with all adopted people, she had two genograms, her adoptive family and her birth family. In her case, as with many adoptees, one was known and the other was completely unknown. The adoptee's task is to consolidate the two families into a sense of personal identity. This is difficult to do when there is little knowledge about and no experience with one of the families.

These issues are particularly salient for adolescents and young adults as they are so involved in establishing who they are (Kornitzer, 1971; Sorosky et al., 1977). It is not infrequent that adoptees identify with and translate into their own lives what little information they do have about their birth parents.

In the case of Sharon discussed above, her family came for therapy because Sharon was acting out sexually. After learning she was adopted and that her birth parents had been college students, the family therapist asked how old her birth mother had been when she was born. When the parents replied "19," the therapist turned to Sharon and said "what's your hurry, you've got four years." The parents' response was first surprise, then laughter. Sharon looked angry at first and then she struggled to control a secret smile. It was clear that Sharon was identifying with the one thing she knew about her mother. The family's planned trip to the agency was in part an effort to gain more information so Sharon's birth parents could be defined more fully than a couple of college kids who got pregnant.

The powerful wish to search among adoptees undoubtedly has many sources (Schechter and Bertocci, 1990) and one very important one is the need to consolidate identity. Family therapists who have worked in the Bowen model of family of origin work find that the adoptee's need to search and the benefits in that for the searcher are very congruent with family of origin practice. in family of origin work, the goal is to reconnect with family members who have been out of contact, surface the secrets, become a student of the family of origin, learn about the salient events, family themes and expectations and make a person-to-person relationship with every member of the family system (Bowen, 1978; Hartman and Laird, 1983).

Although the adoptee's goals may be more modest, the goal of the search is to in some way reconnect with origins, hopefully make a personal connection with the parents, and gain some information about the biological family. Schechter and Bertocci (1990), reporting on their research on adoptees who have searched, write "Adoptees typically comment on the part of me that's missing, and on the desire to 'find out who I really am,' to 'learn my true identity'" (p. 80).

When seeing an adult adoptee in clinical practice, the issue of the search should be a part of the therapy. Whether to search, of course, is a highly personal decision. Readiness varies a good deal and many adoptees choose never to search.

For most adoptees, whether they want to try to find their birth parents or not, referral to an adoptee group can be very helpful. This, in itself, helps the adoptee feel connected, feel less different, less isolated. As one adoptee said, "Finding other adoptees was like finding my brothers and sisters." Through participation in such groups, the meaning of being an adoptee, the individual's identity as an adoptee is clarified and elaborated. Also, as with birth mothers, self-esteem is enhanced and adoptees, who have been the most disempowered in the adoption triangle, become empowered through joining with others in advocating for their rights and for the reform of adoption practice.

For those who wish to search, the support and help of their fellow adoptees is crucial. Beginning a search can be a frustrating, disappointing and disempowering experience. In most states, records are sealed and it takes enormous ingenuity, creativity, and dogged detective work to overcome the many obstacles to the search. In fact, sharing stories of the search process and of how the obstacles were overcome is very much a part of adoptee groups. The search story is, in a sense, another chapter of the adoption story but the search story is one of power rather than helplessness, of acting in one's own behalf, of taking charge.

Many social agencies and social workers in states where there is some access to information about the adoptees' origins, recommend that the adoption agency act as a mediator in the search process, doing the search for the adoptee, contacting the birth parent and making whatever arrangements seem appropriate.

Many adoptees feel this is not a satisfactory approach because the search itself, going through all the work, is an important part of the healing process. In assuming a mediating role, the agency is again in charge, as it was at the time of the adoption, and again places the adoptees in a passive role. The adoptees' view that they should do their own search is supported by family therapists' experience in family of origin work. In this model of therapy, the therapist acts as coach and gives encouragement and support, but the work is done by the client. The value lies, at least in part, in the fact that they are doing this for themselves. As one adoptee said after she completed her search, "I feel so wonderful that I have done this for myself. It is like giving myself a gift, a wonderful gift."

CONCLUSION

Every clinician is in post-adoption practice. Unfortunately, many of the clients we see have suffered in part because of the policies of traditional adoption practice. Such practice has been built on secrecy and on the denial of the real differences between adoption and biological parenting. Adoptees, birth parents, adoptive parents, and professionals are joining together to reform adoption practice, to work toward a range of models of openness in adoption. Some adoption experts are taking the position that open adoption should be the standard (Pannor and Baran, 1984) and any move toward closure must be justified in the individual case. It is hoped that in the future fewer members of the adoption triangle will suffer from the iatrogenic effects of secrecy and denial.

Efforts are also underway in many states to open adoption records, at least at the point when an adoptee attains maturity. To date, this effort has been unsuccessful in most states but adoption groups and others concerned about the right of adoptees to the information the rest of us take for granted continue to work to change the laws. Such a change would make the search for biological family much easier for those who wish to follow this course. It would also affirm for adoptees that their wishes are valid and that they should have the same rights as others to know their parents.

Even as these issues are slowly being resolved, clinicians will be serving a whole new group of adoptees and their families, adoptees who have lost family and homeland, the thousands of children who have been adopted through international programs in South America and Asia. We do not know too much about these children or how they will fare, but we must be ready to hear their stories and to learn from them as we have learned from adoptees, birth parents, and adoptive parents in the past decade.

NOTES

1. Estimates of the number of adoptees in the United States run as high as four million. As many adoptions are unreported, an exact count is not possible to obtain.
2. Throughout this discussion, the focus will be on birth mothers. A very large percent of the birth parents who have become involved in the birth parent movement are women. There is growing interest in the birth father and a move to protect his rights. As yet, however, few birth fathers have come forward, little is known about their experience.

REFERENCES

Bowen, Murray (1978). *Family therapy in clinical practice*. New York: Aronson.
Brodzinsky, D. & Schechter, M.D. (1990). *The psychology of adoption*. New York: Oxford.
Carlsen, Mary Baird (1988). *Meaning-making: The therapeutic processes in adult development*. New York: Norton.
Deykin, E.Y., Campbell, L. & Patti, P. (1984). The post-adoption experience of surrendering parents. *American Journal of Orthopsychiatry*, 54, 271-280.
Hartman, A. & Laird, J. (1983). *Family centered social work practice*. New York: Free Press.
Hartman, A. & Laird, J. (1990). Family treatment after adoption: Common themes. In D. M. Brodzinsky and M. D. Schechter (Eds.), *The psychology of adoption*. New York: Oxford University Press.
Kirk, H.D. (1964). *Shared fate*. New York: Free Press.
Kornitzer, M. (1971). The adopted adolescent and the sense of identity. *Child Adoption*, 66, 43-48.
Laird, J. (1989). Women and stories: Restorying women's self constructions. In M. McGoldrick, C.M. Anderson and F. Walsh (Eds.), *Women in families*. New York: Norton.
Pannor, R. & Baran, A. (1984). Open adoption and standard practice. *Child Welfare* 63(3), May-June, 245-250.
Paul, N.L. & Grasser, G. (1965, Winter). Operational mourning and its role in conjoint family therapy. *Community Mental Health Journal*, I, 339-345.
Schechter, M.D. & Bertocci, D. (1990). The meaning of search. In D.M. Brodzinsky and M.D. Schechter (Eds.), *The psychology of adoption*. New York: Oxford University Press.

Sorosky, A., Baran, A., & Pannor, R. (1975). Identity conflicts in adoptees. *American Journal of Orthopsychiatry.* 45, 18-27.

Sorosky, A., Baran, A., & Pannor, R. (1984). *The adoption triangle.* New York: Doubleday.

Stern, Daniel (1985). *The interpersonal world of the infant.* New York: Basic Books.

Wasson, V. P. (1939). *The chosen baby.* Philadelphia: Lippincott.

Winkler, R. & van Keppel, M. (1984). *Relinquishing mothers in adoption: Their long term adjustment.* Monograph #3. Melbourne: Institute of Family Studies.

Shame and Violence:
Considerations in Couples' Treatment

Dennis Balcom

INTRODUCTION

Rick described splintering their bedroom door in his violent rage. He had felt dismissed by Becky. He felt inadequate to satisfy her expectations. When he feels this way his typical pattern is to scream, rage, throw objects and hit Becky. In recounting these events, Rick avoided looking at me.

The central position of this paper is that shame is a crucial dynamic in addressing the issue of wife abuse. Social workers and family therapists often deal with couples in which men are violent against their female partners. Often, these treatments end in crisis, without positive resolution of the couple's difficulties.

Wife abuse engenders shame for victim and perpetrator. Men who batter strive to hide their sense of inadequacy behind their violence. Battered women experience shame through their inability to escape. Yet shame in the arena of couples therapy, remains largely unexplored by social workers and family therapists. I believe shame is a critical concept in understanding and treating the problems which arise in all couples therapy where wife abuse in an issue.

Combining the concept of shame with the problem of wife abuse broadens and deepens our perspective and efficacy. Coupling an understanding of the dynamics of shame and of abuse leads to a more complex understanding of male violence.

This paper will address the interaction of shame and violence in couples. I will present definitions of shame, types of shame cycles, and how

Dennis Balcom, MSW, ACSW, BCD, is in private practice in Cambridge, MA. Correspondence can be sent to 240 Concord Ave., #2, Cambridge, MA 02138.

shame effects male development. The treatment section focuses on four distinct stages.

SHAME AND VIOLENCE

Theories about shame are still speculative and under development. The dynamics of shame continue to elude theorists and clinicians, although several authors have undertaken the task of clarification. Wurmser (1981), Lewis (1971) and Morrison (1989) discuss shame from a psychoanalytic viewpoint. Kaufman (1985, 1989) bridges the intrapsychic and the interpersonal arenas of shame. Fossum and Mason (1986), Potter-Efron (1989) and Potter-Efron and Potter-Efron (1987) address the interface of shame and addictions. These shame theorists provide some of the theoretical basis for this paper. Shame emanating from violence comes from a variety of sources; individual development, male socialization, interactional patterns and in the couple, and sometimes the treatment itself. Violence includes acts of physical harm, verbal threats, and psychological terrorism. The primary focus of treatment is on the cessation of violence concurrent with the exploration of shame experiences. Throughout this paper 'men' will refer to the cohort of men who have the dual issues of shame and violence. Their "female partners" include legally married wives, live in partners, and lovers.

DEFINITIONS OF SHAME

Shame, in its simplest sense is a judgment of the self as worthless, inadequate, devalued by the self and others. Shame is innate and accessible throughout the life span (Tompkins, 1987). It is both an affect and a character attribute or style.

Normal shame, as an affect, passes with the immediate experience. Accurate self judgment is one experience of normal shame. Failure includes a negative self judgement. One example might be a low grade on an examination. The cause of the low grade might be an inability to conceptualize the material. A student with positive self esteem will normally feel bad (a sense of failure or shame) for receiving a low grade. The experience will pass with time as the student masters the material. Accurate self judgment is reality oriented. When shame is a character attribute, the student has a distorted belief that one low grade equals a "bad student" forever. Normal shame, as experienced in accurate self judgement, does not cause a person to become shame bound.

Illuminating a deficiency in a person triggers shame. The deficiency, real or imagined, is always about the fundamental worth of the person. The experience of shame, either as affect or character style, precipitates inaccurate judgments of the self as worthless. Various words convey the sense of worthlessness: bad, poisonous, rotten, failure, no good, inadequate, incompetent. The overall judgment which flows from the feeling of worthlessness is that the person has always been and will always be this deficient character.

Shame as a core of personality dramatizes the experience of worthlessness. A person with shame imbedded in his or her character experiences mistakes or failures as the total devaluation of self. Shame in relation to violence belongs in this realm of character attributes or styles.

Kaufman (1989) distinguishes three types of shame. One is *the experience of normal shame*. In this definition, a person experiences the blush of shame, the hot flush passes quickly and does not reflect on one's self worth. Normal shame ordinarily does not led to violence.

Internalized shame, Kaufman's second description, occurs when one incorporates shame as a personality attribute. The primary way this occurs is through an identification with the shaming caretaker. A shaming caretaker will berate a child for having needs or feelings. This identification leads the child to develop a self image as unworthy, bad or toxic to others. The child might show this as avoidance, shyness, or mortification. Shame can limit the child's options to the point of constricting her or his social development throughout life.

Shame bound, Kaufman's third definition, occurs in the same manner as internalized shame. The major difference is that it becomes the central attribute around which the person's personality or character becomes structured. The internalized shame becomes the sole identity from which to view the world. For shame bound people, every social experience and description of the self has a core of shame. Shame truly disables these individuals.

A person who is *shame bound* or who has *internalized shame* is at risk to be in an abusive relationship. Obviously, not all individuals with shame issues become violent or victims of violence. However, the converse, is much more likely to be true; perpetrators and victims of violence have shame issues.

BECOMING SHAME BOUND

How does one become shame bound or take on internalized shame? Three processes occur in children that cause shame to become problematic.

The first process is direct shaming actions or statements. A child forms his or her self image through the process of identification. The child's self image depends upon how important people relate to her or him. Verbal statements which limit or silence the child's needs, feelings, or drives lead to shame. A child believes what parents tell, show, or teach. Parents who are verbally and physically abusive instill shame in their children.

The indirect process of neglect is the second method by which children become shame bound. This includes the absence or neglect of adequate attention to the growing child's needs, drives, and desires. Neglect fosters in the growing child feelings of worthlessness, hopelessness, and despair. For many children in these types of families, the quest is for physical and psychological survival. A chronically drunk parent is unable to feed the children, help with homework, and provide a nurturing bedtime ritual.

Another example of an indirect process of a profoundly shaming event is incest, or any other severe abuse. Incest is abusive to children by violating their emotional and physical boundaries. Its only function is to gratify the distorted desires of the older relative. It teaches children that they exist solely to satisfy the relative's needs.

The third process is the intergenerational transmission of shame. Shame children mature as shame bound adults. Through socialization in a shame based family they are blind to respectful ways of relating to themselves and others. As adults they are at risk of selecting a mate who is shaming or dealing with his or her own shame issues. They perpetuate the intergenerational transmission of shame by shaming others as a defense.

The targets for their defensive shame are spouses and children. Defensive shaming seeks to avoid acknowledging one's inadequacies by dominating another. Displacement is one device through which this occurs. The common story of a man dominated by his supervisor at work, who comes home and kicks the dog, is an example. A shame bound man seeking to avoid shame will project it onto accessible others, primarily those dependent or subordinate to him.

Male Socialization And Shame

Men and women experience shame in all of these categories. By virtue of socialization and gender, I suggest that the experience of shame differs for men and women. This section will address how shame is part of male socialization.

Lewis (1971) suggests that women are more shame prone, while men are more likely candidates for guilt. My clinical experience does not support her position. More recent research demonstrates that men are more shame-prone and that shame proneness correlates positively with dependency (Mirman, 1984). This correlation with dependency fits the profile for abusive men as well.

Shaming is one primary method of male socialization. Families and society teach boys to be tough, to harden themselves to feelings, and to treat their bodies as machines. Expressing emotional or physical vulnerability results in shaming. Peers, fathers, uncles, older brothers express ridicule when boys express pain, fear, sadness, dependency or a need for nurturance. Male socialization encourages boys to engage in violence in both the family and the community. I recently overheard a group of preschool boys; "Let's kill Mary." shouted one. Another responded "No, let's just scare her."

"Boys will be boys," grants permission for brothers to fight painful battles without parental help. Bullying larger brothers silence their sisters' voices. Boys become both perpetrators and victims of violence in these instances.

Boys enter a frightening world of mastery before they have the psychological or physical development to succeed. Boys, rewarded for hiding vulnerability, become men who enter a frightening emotional world without adequate preparation and with exactly the wrong kind of training. A frightening adult task for men is that of intimate relationships. Many men learn to fear closeness, yet because they are human, they seek it. The result is a struggle in which men can only tolerate relationships through denial of dependency. Dependency, a basic human need, becomes equated with weakness. Men emphasize accomplishments not emotion, so when a woman desires emotional relating, it perplexes and intimidates them.

Male bonding often focuses on rejecting and devaluing women. If we accept the argument and evidence that male socialization is instrumental rather than expressive, it logically follows that men would devalue expressiveness. Men find it insurmountable to reconcile the female message of expressiveness with the male message to hide vulnerabilities. "Don't be a sissy." "Only girls cry." "Stop acting like a girl." These are messages many men had pounded into them as boys.

These messages serve a doubly destructive purpose. First they deny boys access to their full range of feelings. Second they instruct boys to scorn girls. Boys who take on these messages persist as adults in treating women as unappreciated objects (Luepnitz, 1988).

Men, socialized to define their worth and masculinity through autonomy and mastery, will experience shame (a basic sense of inadequacy) when unable to succeed in these quests. They are susceptible to conflicts in two relationship domains.

The first domain is when their female partners ask, urge, or demand that they perform better in relationships. These requests from female partners are typically about emotional expressiveness. It feels unmasculine, even annihilating, to men when asked to become more like their female partners.

A husband might perceive his wife's request for closeness as a statement that he is not performing well and is therefore bad or inadequate. This feeling of shame, when aroused, can lead to violence as a method of regaining autonomy. By dominating the woman, the violence restores equilibrium for the man, who is then able to regain his sense of autonomy or mastery.

The second domain is the disowned aspects of the man's dependency needs. Yet men do have dependency needs which they are unable to satisfy except in the context of a loving relationship. These needs include all their partners' requests: more emotional expressiveness other than anger, tenderness towards her and the children, affection which does not lead to sex, and a softening of his body armor. Men may code their dependency needs in ways that do not automatically make sense to their partners. For example, adolescent boys who want to be close to girls often hit them. An adolescent girl does not know that this is the boy's inappropriate attempt to convey his attraction to her.

The adult male equivalent of this is the use of sexual innuendo or bravado. Instead of bring a woman closer as he desires, it offends and distances her.

Successful fulfillment of adult dependency needs requires a high tolerance of frustration, since no one will be consistently able to respond adequately to quell his or her inner fears of deprivation. Shame bound men lack the capacity to tolerate this normal frustration, which leads to abusive behavior. They seek immediate gratification of their hunger, sex drive, or demands, masking their underlying dependency needs in disguised forms.

SHAME CYCLES

Shame operates in cycles on the individual, couple, and treatment system levels. Shame cycles are recursive and persistent. Recursive refers to cycles which are self regenerating and repetitive. These persistent qualities repel bids to stop or change them. All cycles have variations which provide openings for interventions.

Individual Shame Cycle

One individual shame cycle is the *control release* cycle described by Fossem and Mason (1986, p. 13).

> Each position on the cycle supports and intensifies the other position. The release phase, either by its chaotic nature or its violation of the control values, adds to the shame. The control phase feels like a refuge from shame, but is actually only a hiding place and covers the shame.

The control release cycle seeks to avoid the feeling of shame during the control phase. The abuse which occurs through loss of control in the release phase engenders shame. Upon experiencing shame, a person will seek to regain control to avoid the flood of affect. For individuals with internalized shame or who are shame bound, it is self perpetuating. The trigger for this cycle might be an internal stimulus, such as a thought which leads to feeling shame, or an external stimulus such as contempt from another.

Couple's Shame Cycle

Each member of the couple will experience his or her individual shame cycle. Together they construct a relationship shame cycle. The ways in which each strives to defend him or her self against experiencing shame or vulnerability precipitates shame in the other (Nathanson, 1987).

Lansky (1987) identifies five stages in the couple's shame cycle which can lead to violence. First he sees a *tendency towards personality disorganization*. Both partners are susceptible to regression (personality disorganization) during the best of times. During times of stress, heightened regression occurs. This includes "a neediness and a shame over it that is not relieved in any useful way by the marital system" (Lansky, 1987, p. 357). Each's effort to diminish the chaotic state resulting from the disorganization fail to cover the vulnerabilities. Next comes a *precipitant* to the acts of violence, which might simply be a bad mood or minor disagreement. The *prodrome* phase is the emotional awareness that immediately precedes the violence, often experienced as confusion or persecutory.

The *act* of violence, which Lansky (1987) sees as impulsive, occurs and then leads to more shame for both partners. *Reactions* to the violence comprise the final step. Guilt and shame might be part of this reaction.

Upon entering the prodrome phase of a shame cycle, battering becomes almost inevitable. During this phase, an erosion of conflict resolution skills occurs. Couples have trouble maintaining a positive connection.

Simultaneously, the woman is also experiencing disorganization. Threats and abusive behavior weaken her internal resources. She is less competent to protect herself in the crisis. Many women come from families with an abuse history. If they suffer further abuse in an adult relationship the result is ingrained learned helplessness. No matter which way they turn, they do not perceive help to be available.

The individual shame cycle of either partner can trigger the relationship shame cycle. This is not to be misunderstood in regards to the responsibility for violence. The abusive man is still solely responsible for his violence towards his partner. In no circumstances should the therapist allow the man to use his experience of shame, or his defenses against shame, as a justification to batter.

Let's return to our case example to see how these cycles function. For Rick and Becky, each tried to reduce the onslaught of shame by projecting responsibility onto the other. Projection is a typical defense against shame. Each disowned the personal experience of inadequacy, then ascribed the disowned sense of inadequacy to the other. Rick especially felt vulnerable upon returning home from work. He wished that Becky would nurture and feed him as a means to overcome his low self esteem. Her wish was the same, with the chronic fear of not knowing what she would encounter upon coming home. Rick was often enraged or depressed. Would he have dinner ready for her and be able to nourish her? Both had stressful jobs and often felt overwhelmed in accomplishing the daily maintenance tasks for the relationship. Neither believed in the good will of the other or that they would ever have their basic needs met.

Some couples employ shame and violence to regulate emotional distance (Lansky, 1987). Both are high risk methods of finding the right distance, always resulting in the wrong distance. Becky would pull away from Rick during the control phase as a way to protect herself. Rick would experience this as rejection, in which he experienced deep shame. He wondered why she would distance herself and assumed it was because he was a bad person. Defending against this rejection and self definition, Rick moved to the next phase of the cycle. He would verbally attack her, claiming that she was intentionally hurting him. The more he attacked, the more she withdrew.

Predictably, when the bond stretched too thin, they would rebound and reconnect. Usually Becky moved closer to Rick after he was violent. To do this, she had to ignore or suppress the recent threats to her life and the physical damage that she had suffered.

Their basic love and empathy for each other came from recognizing the shared bond of severe childhood wounds. Both covertly wished that the other would be better than their parents in nurturing them. This wish disabled them as adults from implementing other functional solutions for their relationship difficulties. A negative connotation of this wish is "I don't deserve better." A positive connotation of this wish is "We can understand and get better at relating."

As Rick and Becky recognized the different shame cycles, they gained better control over them as individuals. As a couple, their understanding helped reduce the shaming interactions which had infected their daily married life.

Shame Cycles in the Therapeutic System

The third shame cycle resides in the treatment system. Small lapses of empathy by the therapist is one example. An empathic lapse can activate a break in the fragile therapeutic alliance. Clients can feel misunderstood or abused by the therapist and flee from the treatment. For example, the inflection of the therapist's voice might show disinterest in the client. The client could experience this as not being valued by the social worker, feel ashamed, and prematurely terminate.

Second, the social worker may actively shame the client. Any form of clinical abuse, contempt for the client, or boundary violation constitutes active shaming. The most despicable form is when the therapist misuses his or her power by sexually abusing the client.

A third form of shame in the therapeutic system occurs when clients actively attempt to shame the therapist. Comments which seek to devalue are one example. Rick said "Why haven't *you* stopped the violence? I don't think you know how to help us." Frightening postures or threats to leave the therapy session are other disabling and potentially shaming maneuvers. If emotionally wounded in this fashion by a client, a social worker may question her or his own competence.

Finally, a therapist may be struggling with his or her own shame issues. In treating shamed clients, the social worker may vicariously reexperience his or her own painful life events, engendering a sense of incompetence, stagnation, or disempowerment.

SHAME INDUCED BY VIOLENCE

Upon beginning an episode of violence, Rick was aware "Once I've gone over the line the damage is already done. I might as well continue and be violent because I'm afraid of the consequences when its over." Here, Rick is describing his release phase which occurred after a period of being in control, working hard to restrain himself. Unfulfilled needs typically triggered his release phase. The consequences had to do with justice in which he sought to establish a victim and perpetrator balance. He cast Becky in the roles of provoker of his violence and as executioner of his punishment. He tried to excuse his violence by insisting that she was "provocative."

Rather than acknowledge his responsibility for the violence, Rick would project responsibility onto Becky. He would use rage and projection as defenses against his shame. He shouted and threatened, hoping to force her to accept his view of what caused the incident. Usually, this meant that he wanted her to accept responsibility for causing him to be violent.

Another repercussion of his violence was his self criticism. Rick would berate himself for his loss of control, leading to increasingly deeper feelings of despair, worthlessness and hopelessness. These feelings would lead him back to the control part of the shame cycle. He sought to make "points" with Becky by being especially caring and careful with her. Obviously, as long as he continued in the cycle, one phase followed another.

The episodes of violence terrified Becky. Rick's threats against her life enraged her, and she adamantly voiced her wish for him to stop. In her fearfulness she would demand that he leave, that they separate and divorce. He would calm down, apologize and be contrite. She felt ashamed by reverting to their normal interactions; they resumed their daily life together (the couple's control-release cycle). Becky would later say "I feel ashamed that I didn't leave when I could have."

The aftermath was painful for Becky. The most damaging results were the physical and psychological pains inflicted on her. Other results were the erosion of her self esteem and the taking on of a battered wife identity, which reinforced her childhood victim identity. A confirmation of her world view that people deliberately hurt you, and there is no recovery from wounds of this nature was the final consequence.

PROBLEMS IN TREATMENT

Treating couples where abuse occurs can be dangerous (Balcom & Healey, 1990; Pressman, 1989; Stark & Flitcraft, 1988). Clients or therapists under-reporting or minimizing the abuse is the first danger. One explanation is the shame that both abusers and victims feel. The therapist must ask questions to elicit accurate information about the violence.

The therapist may unwittingly act as a stabilizing or homeostatic influence. This is a danger in any therapy. However, in this therapy the danger is greater because the stakes are higher. Wife abuse is difficult to treat. To do effective treatment social workers have to confront their own denial or lack of education on this issue. At times we will feel helpless and not know how to help. It can be frightening to work with abusive men. These factors can lead to problems of not wanting to confront the issues and thereby supporting the status quo.

Overidentification with one member of the couple is an obvious danger at these times. Another is a negative countertransference. Social workers have to be careful not to be reactive to the pain of these couples. If the client's words or actions feel provocative, a wish to retaliate may emerge. This is a warning sign that the social worker senses her or his own shame or vulnerability.

Retaliation is a desire to hurt the person who hurt us. In shame terms, it equates with the desire to expose someone who has exposed us. The shame laden fantasy is that by exposing the other person, I remain hidden and safe. However, the act of retaliation carries with it its own shame. Retaliation replaces adequate self protection, thus perpetuating the shame cycle.

With these problems in mind, and remembering that the woman is more at risk than the man, couples therapy can be viable. The primary reason is that the couple is requesting help in remaining a couple. They enter treatment with neither self improvement nor separation in mind, but with the wish to transform their current relationship. Often, these couples have experienced earlier treatments as failures. The previous therapeutic failures become additional internalizations of shame. The wife may feel ashamed that she stayed or left for a shelter but returned (Aguire, 1985; Gelles, 1976). By identifying battery as the core treatment issue, husbands often feel ashamed as it unmasks their failure of self control.

The criteria for couples work that the violence must first cease makes clinical sense, yet it often does not conform to actual clinical experience. More likely, similarly to substance abuse treatment, there will be periods of remission followed by episodes of violence while the treatment progresses.

Each social worker or family therapist will make an individual decision on the best approach to these dangers. Some will elect not to do couples treatment under any circumstances. Others will engage couples while violence is occurring. Information about the shameful hidden aspects of violence can facilitate this often agonizing decision.

The frustrating nature of the treatment often injures the social worker's self esteem. To counteract the shame inducing effects these couples have on the therapist, regular supervision or consultation may be helpful. Personal psychotherapy is another option if the social worker is repeatedly inducted or stuck.

TREATMENT OF SHAME AND VIOLENCE

Effective treatment results in the cessation of violence. By introducing shame into the formulation of why men batter, a worthwhile expansion of intervention strategies occurs. Most abusive men are not sociopathic sadists. They have ego strengths which the social worker can nurture. Utilizing the ego strengths of men and women occurs in at least four stages of treatment.

Stage One: Therapy Contracts

The initial stage of treatment defines the couple's problems in terms of violence and shame. The formation of therapy contracts takes place in this phase. The primary one is for no violence which ensures the female partner's safety. The second contract is for no shaming which seeks to de-escalate the emotional intensity of the couple.

The question of discontinuing treatment if the violence persists is an important component of the safety contract. The social worker has to specify criteria for deciding when to terminate couples therapy if there is violence.

Unintentionally, the process of establishing contracts raises shame for clients. By identifying the issues of violence and shame, the clients will feel a sense of failure. Sometimes, even asking for help by entering treatment engenders shame.

In forming safety contracts, the social worker clearly states the man's responsibility for the violence. The man typically experiences this confrontation, and the consequences if he breaks the contract. He may feel that the social worker establishes the contract and wields power over him.

If the social worker is a woman, he may feel that she is in a coalition against him. The shame can inhibit treatment by detracting all participants from the primary goal of ending the violence. A couple caught in their shame cycle has little energy or motivation left over to rebuild the relationship.

The above concerns about how difficult it is for these couples to separate or maintain safety will be part of the treatment. Shame automatically gets introduced at this point during the discussion about the details of the violence, safety contract, and consequences. A safety contract might consist of the following elements: cessation of violence, attendance for each in therapy groups, and abstinence from alcohol during treatment.

A no shaming contract that aims at shame reduction and that reduces violence, is the basic therapeutic position. This helps the couple identify how they act in shaming ways. No one wants to experience shame. Therefore the reduction of the experience of shame becomes a powerful motivating force which helps couples find new solutions to their difficulties. Both types of contracts create new boundaries for the couple.

Stage Two: Helping the Couple
Identify Their Shame

In this stage, addressing the individual and couple shame are the primary interventions. The social worker can further explore shame by commenting on clients' lowering eyes, turning away, or using shaming statements. One woman said that when her husband was violent to her, she wanted to disappear, and she wanted him to disappear. This is a shame laden statement (I want to disappear), which provides a springboard for further discussion of the theme. Joel swiveled around in his chair when his wife cried about his abusing her. He did not want to face the pain he had caused her. Bill blamed Mary for his hitting her. This projection of blame illustrated his feeling of inadequacy and inability in emotionally responding to her.

The fundamental treatment of shame seeks to reveal it. By the therapist identifying these signals from clients through the treatment, they eventually become astute at using the language and become self conscious (in a positive way) about their own shame and that of their partner. The therapist's perceptions may make clients feel self-conscious. To do this type of confrontation in an empathic manner, the therapist or social worker has to believe that clients will ultimately benefit from the exploration and revelation of their shame.

Uncovering the Wounds of Shame

Shame bound people use defense and secrecy to hide their shame, yet exposing the hiding places of shame is the therapeutic task. The process of exposure is akin to ripping of a bandage to inspect an infected wound. To see and cure the wound requires removing the bandage. Shame is an emotional or psychological wound that the client does not want to acknowledge. The client hides behind the defenses (bandages) of denial, minimization, rage, contempt, and projection of responsibility. Removing the bandage actually hurts, and the patient is rightfully apprehensive about the underlying wound. As health care professionals, we know that wounds can heal. Some pain in treatment is usually necessary to effect the cure. Being free from this wound allows the shame bound person to experience shame as a normal affect.

Uncovering the clients' wounds need to be done with care. It is respectful to uncover it, since the client is asking for help. One respectful method to insert the concept of shame is to share with the client the dilemma presented above. The social worker can say that they have an important way to understand the client's experience. "The feelings or reactions you might have as we do this concern me." The client should not get the idea that something bad or wrong is happening in the treatment because they are feeling uncomfortable. I explain their discomfort as a necessary part of the process and a sign of progress.

Another approach is the use of relabeling. Relabeling simply means giving a different label to the feeling or behavior. A violent man might say he feels guilty. Guilt originates from violating a moral precept. Shame revolves around a sense of personal inadequacy. By exploring in detail his description of his feeling, an accurate relabeling becomes possible. Clients frequently resonate to this shift in label, at which point they are open to further exploration of shame. Of course, a client may experience both shame and guilt from the same behavior.

Interpretation of shame as an intervention carries the risk of rewounding the client. The therapist presents to the client something which the client is not yet conscious. The accuracy of the interpretation may feel too revealing for the client. All interpretations pose a narcissistic injury to the client.

Shame about shame is likely; therefore, the therapist needs to maintain a delicate balance to convey acceptance while continuing to address the issues of shame and violence.

In working with shame the social worker has to attend to the maintenance and restoration of empathy. Clients give clues that they feel injured; eventually they need to acknowledge responsibility for their feelings. Yet early in the treatment they do not have methods of doing this, so it is the therapists' responsibility. Later, the client and therapist can share that responsibility.

Stage Three: Identifying and Transforming Shame Defenses

In the third stage of treatment the task is to help the client experience *normal* shame as described earlier. Identifying defenses and vulnerabilities reveals the deeper layers of shame, such as Kaufman's (1985) *shame bound* or *internalized shame*. This is the time to include vulnerability contracts. Forming a contract which identifies each partner's vulnerabilities helps interrupt the shame/violence cycles. Each partner identifies her or his own "buttons" and ways to behave differently at those times. I balance the process by having each partner identify and contract for change. The importance of this balance lies only in the shame each carries; the partners are not coequals in the causes or acts of violence. This contracting offers another safe alternative to the violence while addressing shame.

A resocialization or enhancement of coping and defense mechanisms occurs as each partner identifies personal struggles. The witnessing of the other's corrective struggle is useful as a method of increasing empathy and decreasing shame.

Establishing that violence has ceased is difficult to verify. Men may stay in denial about the various ways they persist in dominating. Women who remain in these relationships are at risk as men relapse or normalize their abusive behaviors.

Stage Four: Enhancing the Relationship

The final stage of treatment for couples is enhancing their relationship. Careful monitoring can prevent relapses into old behavior. The new coping mechanisms need supporting. Couples may elect to stop therapy at this point, since the initial problem of violence has abated.

For those couples who choose to continue in therapy, this phase focuses on enhancing communication, conflict resolution, problem solving and intimacy. The therapist can employ different theories and techniques of couples therapy now, as with a nonviolent couple. Finally, of course, is the process of termination.

CONCLUSION

Not all shame based people are violent, but for many, recursive cycles of shame can induce violence. A man who uses violence to defend against his sense of inadequacy deepens his core sense of shame rather than alleviating it. This defense enables the man to hide or deny his inadequacy. A much better solution for all is stopping the violence while addressing the underlying shame. Shame acts as both a feeling and as an imbedded character style.

Shame deepens our understanding for treating violence in couples. Treatment begins with the introduction of shame while establishing safety contracts, with the goal of cessation of violence. The second stage consists of a deeper exploration of shame as a way to understand the cycle of violence and its resulting shame. In the third stage of treatment, each partner becomes less shame bound and shaming through their increased self awareness. This is a prerequisite to satisfactory functioning for the couple. The final stage of treatment seeks to improve the overall couple's relationship.

Shame is also an important concept in understanding ways in which social workers can get disabled in treating couples where there is violence against women.

REFERENCES

Aguire, B. (1985). Why do they return? Abused wives in shelters. *Social Work*, 30, 350-354.

Balcom, D., & Healey, D. (1990). The context for couples treatment of wife abuse. In N. Mirkin, (Ed.), *The social and political contexts of family therapy*. Boston: Allyn & Bacon, 121-137.

Fossum, M., & Mason, M. (1986). *Facing shame: Families in recovery*. New York: Norton & Co.

Gelles, R. (1976). Abused wives: Why do they stay? *Journal of Marriage and The Family*, 38, 659-668.

Kaufman, G. (1989). *The psychology of shame*. New York: Springer Publishing Co.

Kaufman, G. (1985). *Shame: The power of caring*. Cambridge, MA: Schenkman Publishing Co.

Lansky, M. (1987). Shame and domestic violence. In D. Nathanson, (Ed.). *The many faces of shame*. New York: Guilford Press.

Lewis, H. (1971). *Shame and guilt in neurosis*. New York: International Universities Press.

Luepnitz, D. (1988). *The family interpreted: Feminist theory in clinical practice*. New York: Basic Books.

Mirman, M. (1984). *Shame and guilt: Activators, associated unconscious dangers, and defenses*. Unpublished Doctoral Dissertation. Michigan State University.

Morrison, A. (1989). *Shame, the underside of narcissism*. Hillsdale, NJ: The Analytic Press.

Nathanson, D. (1987). Shaming systems in couples, families, and institutions. In D. Nathanson, Ed.). *The many faces of shame*. New York: Guilford Press.

Potter-Efron, R. (1989). *Shame, guilt and alcoholism*. New York: The Haworth Press, Inc.

Potter-Efron, R., & Potter-Efron, P. (1987). (Eds). The treatment of shame and guilt in alcoholism counseling, *Alcoholism Treatment Quarterly*, Vol. *4*, (2).

Pressman, B. (1989). Wife-abused couples: The need for comprehensive theoretical perspectives and integrated treatment models. *Journal of Feminist Family Therapy*, 1, 23-43.

Stark, E., & Flitcraft, A. (1988). Personal power and institutional victimization: Treating the dual trauma of woman battering. In F. Ochberg, (Ed). *Post-traumatic therapy and victims of violence*. New York: Brunner/Mazel.

Tompkins, S. (1987). Shame. In D. Nathanson, (Ed.). *The many faces of shame*. New York: Guilford Press.

Wurmser, L. (1981). *The mask of shame*. Baltimore, Maryland: Johns Hopkins University Press.

Mental Health Services—2001: Serving a New America

Myrtle Parnell
Jo VanderKloot

INTRODUCTION

In that fictional game, nothing remains stable for very long because everything is alive and changing around the player [an all too real condition for many clinicians]. The mallet Alice uses is a flamingo, which tends to lift his head and face in another direction just as Alice tries to hit the ball. The ball, in turn, is a hedgehog, another creature with a mind of its own. Instead of lying there waiting for Alice to hit it, the hedgehog unrolls, gets up, moves to another part of the court and sits down again. The wickets are card soldiers, ordered around by the Queen of Hearts, who changes the structure of the game seemingly at whim by barking out an order to the wickets to reposition themselves around the court.

—Moss-Kantor, 1989

In her description of the Croquet Game in Alice in Wonderland, Rosabeth Moss-Kantor provides us with an apt metaphor for what family therapists experience as the dynamic interaction in the context of a changing world.

We worked in a community agency in the South West Bronx section of

Myrtle Parnell and Jo VanderKloot are adjuncts at New York University School of Social Work and Smith College for Social Work (designated the Lydia Rapaport Lecturers for 1992). The authors are consultants to Bellevue Hospital's Homeless Project; family therapy trainers at Kings County Hospital for Inpatient Adolescent Psychiatry; and co-authors for several chapters and articles on minority issues, poverty and cultural diversity.

The authors are currently under contract to Guilford Press for a book on service delivery in a pluralistic society.

New York City. The area is well known nationally for its poverty, disease, and social problems. It is certainly one of the more drug infested, AIDS infested, and violent parts of the country. Fear is a powerful component of daily life for people of all ages. Those living in wealthy suburban cities read about this environment but do not think of it as related to themselves. However, even a cursory look at the decline of once stable communities suggests that there is an infection growing in America. While it is starting in the inner cities, it is spreading throughout the country. Therefore, what is happening in the South West Bronx is of crucial importance to all social workers, regardless where they are working. If one can accept the hypothesis that the urban poor are a bell wether for society, one will have a clearer understanding of what to look for and what to do for one's self and one's clients. Following World War II, the black family became increasingly single parented. Therapists defined this behavior as deviant and often recommended and even mandated psychiatric treatment. As we come to the end of this century, when one in every two marriages (Sidel, 1986) ends in divorce, we can see that the deviance was in society, not in the black family.

This article proposes that traditional linear, psychodynamic models of therapy are not as effective as multi-level systemic family therapy for treating the urban poor — those families living in a world of disorganization and chaos. There have been many attempts to find treatment approaches to help troubled individuals but " . . . the philosophy that has dominated our century [today] resembled nothing so much as a severe obsessive-compulsive sitting on his bed tying and untying his shoes because he never quite gets it right" (Temas, 1990). We will present a systemic treatment approach that may end the need for the continual tying and untying in the mental health field. We will first describe Chaos Theory, then present arguments against traditional treatment for this population and conclude with a description of a model of therapy for the urban poor. Clinical examples will punctuate the points made here.

CHAOS THEORY

According to Thomas Kuhn (1970) in *The Structure of Scientific Revolution*, under most circumstances scientists work within a set scientific tradition or paradigm. Kuhn makes the analogy between puzzle solving and normal science. Normal scientists do not question the theory under which they are working. The underlying assumptions are accepted. Any anomalies that may occur are put aside or considered bad research. When the anomalies become so numerous, they lead the revolutionary scientists to challenge the underlying assumptions and to develop a new paradigm. In the 1970s, the Chaos scientists (Gleick, 1987) began to emerge, albeit slowly, and influence other disciplines in the hard and social sciences. In recent years, family systems theory has been influenced by the thinking of these scientists. Family therapy practice has grown in its application to white, middle and upper middle income families, but up to now it has had only limited application in the public mental health sector. We believe the time for this shift is ripe and necessary as the problems we face on all levels require a different kind of thinking.

What then is Chaos Theory? To some, it is a science of "process rather than state, of becoming rather than being" (Gleick, 1987). This science breaks across all disciplines because it is a science of the global nature of systems. It is the science of disorder, of all that has been left out. It has an eye for pattern and a taste for randomness and complexity. Chaos theory teaches how to employ the laws that govern complex systems. It deals with the relationships of the parts to the whole.

In order for social workers to feel successful in their work with increasingly difficult families, we would like to suggest a framework for looking at poor families. We will do that by using Al Scheflin's model of levels of intervention (1981). In Figure 1 the circles radiate inward from the nation to the state, community, family, couple and individual. For most poor families these systems have a daily and powerful impact; their whole lives appear to be chaotic. The boundaries of all of these systems are permeable. For most poor families these systems have a daily and powerful impact because they are dependent upon them for survival. In a stable environment it is normally sufficient to address the individual/family unit, assuming a degree of constancy and stability in the larger systems sphere. This is not a realistic assumption in the urban centers of the United States. We will briefly describe these larger systems, zeroing in on an effective way to work with the most difficult clients social workers are seeing with overwhelming frequency.

In the course of our work we have come to appreciate Chaos Theory (Gleick, 1987) as a more useful paradigm for understanding the complexity of interactions and constant change within a societal context. This Theory can be seen as systems theory applied to the widest context. Beginning with the national level, we will provide examples of chaos across systems.

At the national level, we can no longer deny that our institutions are not adequately performing the functions for which they were designed, including the legal system, government, medical and mental health systems,

Figure 1

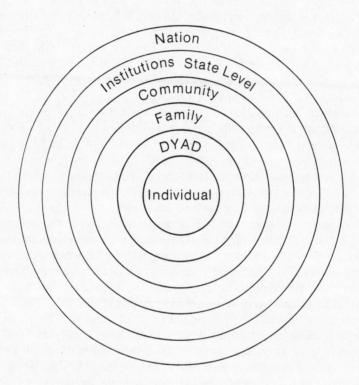

Adapted from Levels of Intervention, 1981
Scheflin, A., M.D.   New York: Brunner-Mazel.

education, and most importantly, the family itself. All of this is occurring
at a time when the federal budget deficit is at an all time high. Part of the
solution to the fiscal crisis has been to target social programs for cuts and
to blame the poor for their poverty. This has created a climate in which
that population is increasingly stressed by both the threat to economic
survival and the negative attitude of society.

On the second level, we hear that the states are also operating in a
deficit mode. Lack of funding even for police is a critical problem for
poor communities; people live in fear for their lives and those of their
children as drive-by shootings and random violence increase. Our public
medical system is so overloaded that hospital beds are in short supply;
patients have to be kept in emergency rooms for days before admission is

possible. AIDS, homelessness, and drug addiction add to already overburdened facilities. Community agencies are confronted with the effects of massive social breakdown and the skills professionals have acquired are not up to the task of solving the problems they face. Mental health agencies, in an effort to avoid burn out, do so by defining the problems they can treat in a narrower and narrower band, creating ever greater problems for emergency rooms.

On the community level, we see the breakdown of the social supports, such as the church or extended family, that have traditionally been the mainstay of the poor black and hispanic communities. Homelessness and relocation have further splintered the ability of poor people to sustain and protect themselves. People do not look out for each other in the streets because they are fearful of being shot. When these kinds of supports give way, it is difficult for families to survive.

What is the impact of this social breakdown on the family? One in four American children lives in poverty (Moynihan, 1986). In urban centers like New York City, one in two children is poverty stricken (Moynihan, 1986). Female headed households, which have grown by 90% in the past five years, account for 53.9% of the families living in poverty (Sidel, 1986). The divorce rate of couples married in the last fifteen years is one in two (Sidel, 1986). As a result many couples choose to remain unmarried. The greatest child killer is poverty, with more children dying of poverty in a five year period than the total American battle deaths in Vietnam (Edelman, 1987).

On the dyadic level, statistics indicate that marriages were failing at a very high rate in the 1970s and early 1980s. Almost 50% of the marriages in this period ended in divorce. The rate was even higher for teenage marriages. For children this often meant that along with the emotional impact of family disruption, there was also a drastic decrease in financial resources available for their care (Sidel, 1986).

On the individual level, there is a serious increase in stress which takes many forms: hypertension, cancer, physical and sexual abuse, and difficulty in job performance.

NEED FOR NEW TREATMENT MODEL

The more popular treatment models and theories, with their emphases on pathology, are non-systemic and use a diagnostic base that is irrelevant, ineffective and insulting to poor people, particularly people of color. They overlook cultural differences and values and seek to find causes of poor people's problems in their intra-psyche. Extreme poverty and homelessness can affect people's feelings about themselves, make some "crazy" and leave many more feeling helpless, powerless and despairing; this can lead to substance abuse as an escape from their misery.

Although the policy and theory courses taught in the schools of social work include issues of poverty, the social work clinician often remains ill-prepared to help poor clients cope with the problems of economic and physical survival they face each day. One day in a poor, urban, community-based clinic makes one painfully aware of the lack of necessary professional tools. Too often social workers treat each case that comes through the door as an isolated situation, rather than see the broader pattern and intervene in the context of the client's world. Linear, individualized interventions often make no sense to these clients.

By contrast, Chaos Theory takes into consideration and validates the totality of the poor person's experience, experience that cannot be understood in a neat, orderly, linear fashion. What poor people do does not fit with our theories about why they do them so we end up blaming people for not doing what we say they are supposed to do, and then wonder why they do not return for appointments or resist our treatment.

How do we recognize pathology in people who are very different from ourselves and who live and survive in a world about which we know little or nothing? How do we distinguish pathology from adaptation? What is a pathological response to living in chaos, a domestic war zone? If we are looking for pathology, we will find it. However, the time has come to use a different lens for understanding poor people. We need to be aware and openly acknowledge how the larger system functions. This is a powerful engagement tool, particularly for those of us who are White working with African-Americans and Latinos. We lack a common ground on which to begin to communicate with people whose frames of reference are very different from our own. It is essential that the middle class clinician makes no assumptions about each client. There are very different ways of being in the world and we do not have a common body of shared knowledge. We must begin as if the person sitting in front of us is from a foreign country and speaks a totally different language. The treatment process, of necessity, must be a collaborative one.

TREATMENT MODEL FOR URBAN POOR

Our treatment model is a non-pathological and inherently respectful of people. Our philosophy combines Chaos Theory (Gleick, 1987) with family systems theory and the work of Milton Erickson (Carter, 1982). It involves four major principles: (1) unconditional positive regard, (2) *OK-'ness*, (3) context, and (4) resistance. We will define each of the four principles and then illustrate them with a clinical example of a mother with two abused daughters.

Unconditional positive regard for the client is the cornerstone of our work with the poor. This means starting with the assumption that people generally do the best they can with the options they perceive are available to them. For example, we have yet to meet two people who came together, had a family, and intentionally tried to make their lives miserable. Most people try to make life better for their children than it was for them growing up. The harder they try, using the only skills and tools they know, the poorer the results and the more likely the escalation of the very behavior they are trying to prevent. They are trying, but they need help in finding a different way. If what people are doing is "not nice," we look for what may be hindering them from being nicer. The uglier the presenting problem, the more necessary unconditional positive regard is to effect a positive outcome regard for the person, not the behavior.

OK'ness, the second principle, deals with the basic integrity of people; people are whole and do not need something added or taken away. Fully implementing this principle requires the solid faith that a person has integrity, even when it appears most lacking. For therapists to accept clients *OK*'ness requires their willingness and flexibility to look for it. Often, it is found where least expected (Carter, 1982).

Our third principle involves paying close attention to the context in which the symptom occurs. This means taking into consideration all parameters that may be impacting on the symptom. It is necessary to look beyond the individual and family. The social environment within the community, state, and even perhaps the country (see Figure 1) may be part of the context that maintains the symptom. It is only if the context is understood that the client's behavior can be fully understood.

Our fourth principle deals with resistance. Some resistance is a normal human reaction to change. However, it often is a client's communication to us that our hypothesis is not complete or that our intervention is unhelpful (Anderson and Stewart, 1983; Imber-Black, 1988; Watzlawick, Weakland, & Fisch, 1974). Resistance may be their only means of protecting themselves from interfering outsiders who do not understand them. In our effort to be helpful, we may forget that resistance is also a normal reaction to change. It is important to look behind the clients' resistance to find a way for them to cooperate in their own treatment in a way that is consistent for them. The more difficult the presenting problem, the more likely social workers are to attempt to push toward a particular direction, out of their own feelings of being overwhelmed. This is just the very time they need to think about this principle. We need to go back to find what we are missing; what do we need in order to include clients in their own treatment so we are working together, not forcing our ideas on them. We agree with Milton Erickson (Carter, 1982) on the importance of fitting clients' needs to the therapy rather than imposing the therapy on them. When people have requested help and feel understood, resistance is usually not a debilitating factor. Understanding this also aids in engaging the involuntary client as well.

Since we do not know what constitutes pathology in a chaotic environment, we emphasize clients' skills and what they are currently doing to function as individuals and members of society. By carefully tracking their behavior, we can understand how they organize their world. We accept their definition of the problem and keep in mind that at one time, that behavior may have been a viable solution to another problem; now, however, it no longer works. For people living on the edge, it may be more productive to enhance their existing skills than to teach them new ones. Identifying their existing skills provides therapists with information that can be used to help clients take charge. Acknowledging and helping them use the skill is empowering for them. Relating to the client as a real, whole person, for whom information and options (not caretaking) need to be provided, gives the message of respect. Most of these people have not had that type of relationship before. This approach increases their self-respect and sense of competency.

Example Demonstrating the Four Principles

Mrs. Jones came to our walk-in clinic stating Children's Protective Services said she had to come in order to get her children back. Both girls had been removed from her home following extensive sexual abuse by her live-in boyfriend. The abuse was medically documented and the boyfriend was sent to jail. Mrs. Jones kept insisting this never happened and she could not understand why no one believed her and why her children were in placement. She also stated she planned to take her boyfriend back when he was released from jail.

It was tempting to argue with her or to brand her "crazy," or both. Instead, the therapist asked her, "What would happen if you were to believe all this to be true?" (This question honored her integrity and said her input was valued). Her immediate response was "I would kill myself!" What initially looked like resistance, now in this context, had a different meaning. This woman's "resistance" to believing the abuse protected her very life. Mrs. Jones was caught in a bind between her need for her boyfriend and her desire to have her children back.

By accepting a person's *OK*'ness, we do not try to get parents to stop their negative behavior as much as we try to get parents to behave in a positive way, making the negative behavior a non-solution to their difficulties, and thereby getting them to stop the abuse. Most people know that abuse is wrong and would do something different if they knew how. The treatment focus must be on stopping the abuse but done in a way that does not offend nor anger, in a way that engages the client. We harness what the client already does well and encourage more of that. In order to track her behavior pattern, to look for existing skills, we explored other situations she had had trouble facing. What emerged was her style of coping, which she had developed in childhood when faced with a situation she felt unable to change. Mrs. Jones had been sexually abused herself as a child and promised herself that when she became a mother, she would protect her children from ever being subjected to that horror. The dilemma was that if she acknowledged the abuse of her children, she would have to acknowledge that she had failed in her promise and her prior solution did not work. With this understanding, the clinical work had a more specific focus on what she could do and revolved around ways she could now protect her daughters, e.g., teaching them what she was learning in treatment about families and about the cycle of secrecy and isolation of incest.

When we work using these basic principles, we are seen by the client as "we" rather than "they." One of our patients (a convicted rapist), when he asked himself what was different in our treatment of him, said, "All the other people were nice and helpful, but it is as if I were out in a canoe in rough water. Everyone else was standing on the shore calling out directions. You dove into the water, swam out, got into the canoe, and showed me a new way to shore" (Parnell & VanderKloot, 1989).

ASSESSMENT

In working with poor families today, it is difficult and often futile, to attempt to prioritize and treat one problem at a time. With the massive breakdown of our social system, as seen in urban centers, each family with so many complex and interweaving problems can seem like a whole caseload. To make an accurate assessment, the clinician must look beyond only the individual family and take into consideration the context in which the family is living. But looking at that context raises important questions. How do you judge the mental health of people living in anarchy, unable to leave, and missing the basic supports necessary for survival? Certainly, one important element of an assessment should consist of looking for the family's existing skills, tracking the perpetual areas of difficulty, and identifying the number and quality of the current or prior helping systems (Imber-Black, 1988).

Two tools that can help identify and organize these and other important elements of a family are genograms (McGoldrick & Gerson, 1985) and eco-maps (Hartman & Laird, 1983). Together they provide an overview of a family, over time, with essential information about their overall functioning, the major unresolved issues, the quality of their relationships, and previously attempted solutions by all involved. This data gathering elicits the individual and family strengths and indicates patterns around which the family is stuck. Both genograms and eco-maps have been described in detail elsewhere. Here, we will only mention the specific use of these tools as they relate to assessment of inner city families.

The genogram (McGoldrick & Gerson, 1985) can be done in a brief form to answer specific questions or in a more comprehensive form covering a range of information, e.g., functioning, relationships, structure, multi-generational issues. It can also be used as an organizing and informative activity for families with young children. Color-coding the genograms (Lewis, 1989) is another useful technique for tracking a particular behavior, incident, or trait through generations.

The eco-map (Hartman & Laird, 1983) gives in diagram form essential information about the many institutions that interface with the family — currently or in the past. It has the additional advantage of providing a quick means of assessing the degree to which the basic needs of the family are being met in a range of areas, and the degree of stress the client is experiencing. An eco-map that shows a family having difficulty negotiating most of the systems they are involved with alerts us to the serious difficulties they are experiencing on so many fronts. Genograms and eco-maps are quick means for gathering a contextual life history, one that is textured with the breadth of a family's interactions and experiences, not a one-dimensional view.*

The following example demonstrates several aspects of a clinical assessment of an urban family struggling with life.

Mrs. Lopez, an obese Catholic/Jewish Hispanic woman, was told to bring her three year old obese daughter, Candida, to the clinic on a weekly basis. Her fourteen year old mildly retarded son, Jose, was already being seen by a therapist for his school misbehavior. Jose scheduled his own appointments and came regularly. However, Mrs. Lopez was erratic in keeping her appointments for Candida.

We are asked to consult with the social worker. In looking for clues to help this family, we reviewed their eco-map (Figure 2). This showed that Mrs. Lopez was involved with six agencies. The broken lines on the eco-

---

*Editor's note: For more on assessments see Tracy and McDonell's article, in this issue.

Figure 2

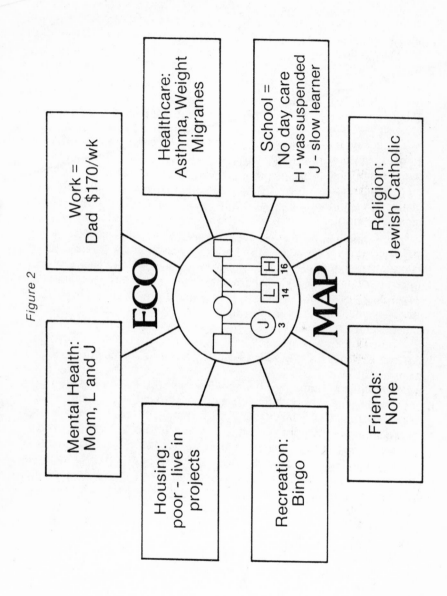

Work =
Dad $170/wk

Healthcare:
Asthma, Weight
Migranes

Mental Health:
Mom, L and J

ECO

School =
No day care
H - was suspended
J - slow learner

Housing:
poor - live in
projects

Recreation:
Bingo

MAP

Religion:
Jewish Catholic

Friends:
None

map indicate systems with which she had difficulty. The only non-conflic-
tual area was bingo. We hypothesized that to work with this family the
social worker needed to understand the process that enabled Mrs. Lopez to
get to bingo regularly. If we could identify this process, we could coach
Mrs. Lopez in using a skill she already had (getting to bingo) in order to
succeed in other areas (getting to the clinic, school and other agencies).
We hypothesized that Mrs. Lopez had someone in the evenings to take
care of the children and drive her to bingo. If that were a correct hypothesis, was the lack of these supports in the daytime related to her inability to
keep her clinic appointments? Using this hypothesis as a starting point, the
social worker could recontact Mrs. Lopez and talk about the logistics of
getting to the clinic. While this seems a minor issue, it often is the simple
aspects that get overlooked. The only one unbroken line on the eco-map
offered a clue to an existing skill that then could be harnessed for other
aspects of her life.

There were many directions we, as consultants, could have taken, e.g.,
the health risk for Candida, Mrs. Lopez's own weight. A good assessment
takes all factors into consideration and then using the eco-map and genogram, finds the connecting patterns, the clues for potential resources, and
existing useable skills. A thorough assessment can short-circuit problems
that might occur later in treatment.

OTHER CONTEXT FOR THE TREATMENT

Working in a "minority" community, it is useful to have at least some
therapists of the same culture or ethnic background as the families being
seen. Since there is an inevitable distrust among different cultures in over-
crowded poor communities, and since there is also a distrust of professionals, having more than a token professional on staff will be most helpful in gaining the communities' trust and cooperation. It is also important
there be a fair representation of both male and female therapists, providing
models for being strong, competent, nurturing and warm men and strong,
competent, nurturing, and assertive women.

In chaotic urban communities, it is helpful to think of appointments in a
more flexible manner. Many clients do not work well with once a week,
fifty minute appointments. Often they do not live by routinized schedules
as do most middle class people; they tend to be focused on a very real and
compelling present rather than the future. Therefore, when we set an ap-
pointment time for some point in the future (e.g. seven days), they may
not show up. We then interpret their "no-show" as their resistance to
therapy, rather than their resistance to our having set an expectation that

does not fit with their life frame. They do, however, work well with encouragement to drop in as needed, which may, or may not be weekly.

Having more than one therapist involved with a family is also advisable, if at all possible. This serves a purpose for the family as well as the therapist. For the family, it gives them a connection to the agency, even if their individual therapist leaves. It is also useful for them to have a number of therapists familiar with their situation so that if they drop in when one is busy, there will be others who know them and can help. For the therapist, working as a team provides mutual emotional support for the very difficult families. The use of one way mirrors for supervision allows for immediate, on-the-spot input and support to the primary therapist.

CLINICAL EXAMPLE OF TREATMENT OF URBAN POOR

In order to illustrate the multi-level complexity of this type of treatment, an example will be used covering the entirety of the treatment. The four principles, the assessment, the importance of the therapist-client relationship, flexibility of therapy frame, the conflictual agendas of helping systems, and the murky termination — all germane to working with this population — will be demonstrated. In the following example, the primary clinician was a Puerto Rican woman who was able to join with this poor, rural, unsophisticated Puerto Rican family in a way that would have been difficult for another therapist. She utilized all the nuances and phrases of rural Puerto Rico that urban, white people probably would not have known. The authors supervised the clinical work and sometimes acted as co-therapists.

Presenting Problem

Maria, age 64, requested medication for her 12 year old grandson, Samuel; she said he was "crazy" and needed tranquilizers. Six years ago, Samuel had been diagnosed, at another clinic, and 25 mgs. daily of Mellaril had been prescribed. Maria increases the medication as she deems necessary. She described Samuel as hyperactive, reported his suicidal gesture at age 8, and said he frequently hallucinates; "he talks to the air." He does have friends, but unfortunately they tend to be older, street smart, and "tough."

The therapist had a drastically different view of Samuel. She described him as a good looking, tall, well developed 12 year old; he was lively, related well and unselfconsciously with adults. Despite poor grades, he seemed of average, if not higher, intelligence. Neither his hyperactivity nor bizarre behavior was evident in the first (or any subsequent) session. The therapist was concerned that Maria used the Mellaril to sedate Samuel, keeping him at home, and restricting his normal activity and interest level.

Family History

Maria, Samuel's paternal grandmother is the primary caretaker for her grandson since Samuel's mother murdered her husband, Maria's son, when Samuel was only a few weeks old. His mother was never apprehended and has since disappeared. Samuel does not know about this murder. Also living in the house is Rosa, age 32, Maria's younger daughter. Rosa has four children, none of whom currently live with her; they are placed out of state with three separate relatives. Rosa has had three nervous breakdowns and has been unable to find permanent employment. Luz, the oldest daughter, is in Florida.

Maria had two husbands; the first is serving a life term for murder in Puerto Rico and the other, whom she met and married in New York, lives in the neighborhood, is an alcoholic, a womanizer, and violent. Maria separated from him because of his physical abuse; it was only through careful questioning that the therapist learned he has remained friendly with Maria, at times lending money and fixing things around the apartment.

Assessment

The family lives in a very poor section of the South Bronx, in housing that is barely inhabitable. The three adults and adolescent boy share a one bedroom apartment which offers no privacy and is in need of major repairs. The apartment has leaks and vermin. The refrigerator frequently malfunctions. The family lives in a neighborhood in which the services — garbage pick-up, police responsiveness, social services, postal service — are minimal. Other community resources, such as activities for children and adolescents, child care, recreation for adults are non-existent. Violence is a daily occurrence.

The genogram of this family (Figure 3) is remarkable in that it reveals four generations of violent men, three of the four having early and violent deaths. Loss and separation issues were powerful emotional inhibitors for this family. A number of women have been abandoned by their own mothers. The family was extremely poor and functionally illiterate over four generations. Until this last generation, no one had completed eighth grade. There are no religious ties, although the family remains culturally

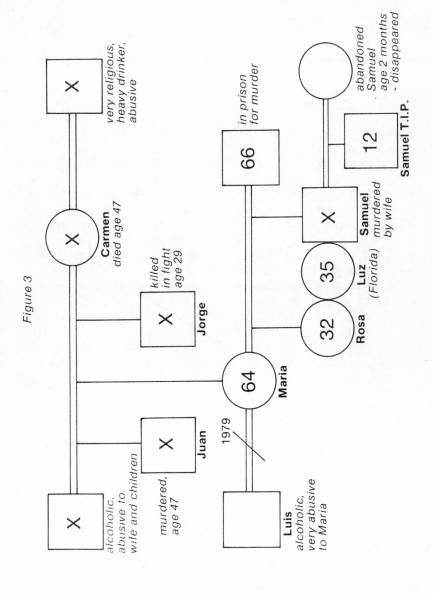

Figure 3

very religious, heavy drinker, abusive

Carmen
died age 47

killed in fight age 29

Jorge

alcoholic, abusive to wife and children

murdered, age 47

Juan

Maria
64

1979

Luis
alcoholic, very abusive to Maria

in prison for murder

66

Rosa
32

Luz
(Florida)
35

Samuel
murdered by wife

abandoned Samuel age 2 months - disappeared

Samuel T.I.P.
12

tied to Puerto Rico. Maria speaks no English, Samuel and Rosa are bi-lingual. The family has very little contact with the American culture other than its institutions—welfare, food stamps, schools and hospitals—all of which they manage very well.

The community ties they have established are adequate to maintain their current level of existence but provide little that would promote economic, social or spiritual growth. Rosa needs to reunite with her children and Samuel needs models for developing into a self-sufficient, competent, young man able to work and care for a family.

Course of Treatment

To organize the volume of information we obtained about this family, we used the genogram and eco-map (see Figures 3 and 4). We searched for a "hook" into the myriad of problems that would help efficiently promote change and make a shift in the family. A basic principle of many schools of family therapy is that one small change may open possibilities for other changes. The most striking characteristic about Samuel's family was its caring for one another so we used their wish and determination to make a better life for themselves as the hook.

After the first session, the team met together and formed the following hypotheses. Maria was a competent woman who had assessed the mental health system and determined that she could best meet her family's financial needs by convincing the school system and the psychiatric system that Samuel was "crazy" and should qualify for social security benefits (SSI). She had previously convinced other health clinics that he needed anti-psychotic medication. We knew that if we challenged that view, she would take Samuel elsewhere for his medication. We also knew that keeping Samuel on medication diminished his chances for a normal adolescence and young adulthood. He would most likely drop out of school, would integrate a self-image of being "crazy," would become increasingly dysfunctional with probable hospitalizations (his aunt had three), and would likely resort to self-medication through street drugs.

We needed to find an intervention that would be both valid for the family and change the context of the presenting problem, while at the same time denying their request to diagnose him psychotic so he would be eligible for SSI. Therefore, at the second session with Maria and Samuel, we presented the following information. We told them that if we declared Samuel crazy, he would be kept at home and cared for by his grandmother who could then protect him from the danger of the streets. They would live off the disability benefits which were superior to welfare. An unfortunate side effect would include his being stigmatized which might hinder

Figure 4

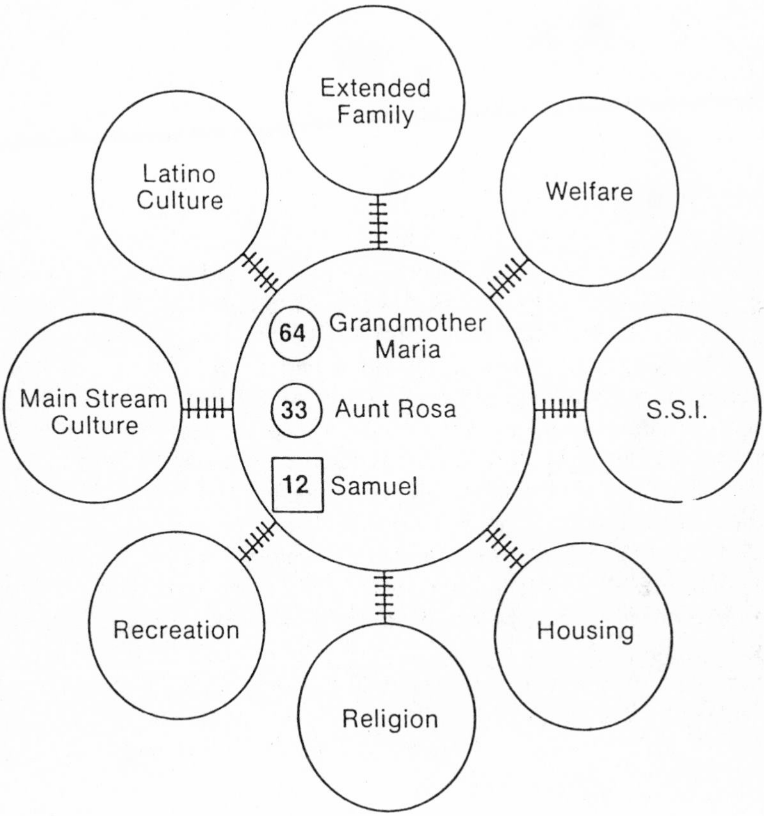

The Samuel Family Eco Map

his personal growth and development. If, on the other hand, we were to declare Samuel well, he would be increasingly exposed to the dangers of the street as he became more and more independent. Maria would make herself sick with worry both for his safety and their financial security. We realized this was a difficult dilemma for the family and for us. We believed Samuel, a bright, attractive and competent, young man, was also aware of this dilemma.

Samuel was delighted with our comments and talked animatedly about things he would like to accomplish when he grows up. Maria, on the other hand was bewildered and visibly shaken. We predicted that the family was in a very difficult bind which would not quickly be resolved. During the process of attempting to resolve their dilemma, we anticipated that Samuel's behavior could conceivably get more bizarre both at home and in school. Maria let us know she clearly got our message that Samuel was not crazy. However, she still needed the disability benefits and needed to protect Samuel. Therefore, she decided to get SSI through another facility and, with us, to participate in family therapy with Samuel and to have him in individual treatment, as needed.

We worked within that parameter and in individual sessions with Samuel, helped him understand his grandmother's concerns while coaching him in ways to meet them without his really being crazy or dysfunctional. At times, this meant he would have to pretend to be crazy; he delighted in colluding with us. He spent a good deal of time scheming crazy ways he might behave in order to get his youngest aunt, who was visiting the family and needed psychiatric care, to see us. He described her as violent and unable to control herself. On two occasions Samuel managed to get both aunts into the medical clinic to meet us.

One of the key family sessions in this evolving process was when we helped Maria tell her grandson about the death of his father and the disappearance of his mother. Maria spoke quietly in a voice choked with emotion as she related the story full of pain that lacked resolution because it was never known how her son really died. Samuel sobbed uncontrollably throughout the remainder of the session, yet he registered relief at knowing what had happened. Maria described his father without denying his shortcomings. Samuel expressed an interest in visiting his father's and uncle's graves. We agreed to have the next session in a cemetery in New Jersey. Samuel called several days later to ask if he could bring his young cousin, his uncle's daughter.

Samuel and his cousin chattered nervously in the car during the hour long trip. They ran out of the car and began reading the different tombstones searching for their fathers. The cousin found her father's grave first and stood there quietly; later she expressed disappointment over the shabbiness and insignificance of the grave site. It was as if she knew that not even in death was it possible to have a decent place to rest. Samuel finally found his father's marker. His stillness as he read his own name on the tombstone (he was a Junior) was in striking contrast to his normal energetic presentation. He said he felt as if he were reading his own tomb. He cried as he told us how he felt standing at the grave of a father he never knew. The ride home was quiet as the two children and Maria were lost in their own thoughts.

The next few sessions dealt with the mourning process. A crucial piece in this work was the careful delineation of how Samuel was like his father and how he was not. It was important for him to know that his life script could be very different. While he physically resembled his father, he was emotionally and intellectually superior to him, even at the age of 12. Grandmother was very clear about this.

As so often happens with these families, the school system, unknowingly, became a force against change. In a ghetto school, where the primary emphasis is often on control and containment, rather than on inquisitiveness and curiosity, an active child like Samuel is sure to be defined as hyperactive, belligerent and disruptive. In fact, Samuel's behavior was a reflection of his being bored in class; that was not understood and he ultimately was placed in a special class for emotionally disturbed children. The school requested an increase in Samuel's medication and Maria complied.

One of the last battles for this family was getting Samuel into a school outside of New York City where he would be less exposed to daily violence, one that had higher intellectual standards. At first the family was adamantly opposed to this idea, but the therapist had an excellent rapport with Maria and was able to get her support and that of the two aunts. Our team psychiatrist reevaluated Samuel and sent a report to the school telling them that there was no psychiatric reason for Samuel to continue in Special Education classes. However, after all of our efforts, we were unsuccessful at getting Samuel into a school outside of the city but at least he was mainstreamed in his current school.

Termination came as it often does with these families. The presenting problems are in remission, and families begin to miss appointments or drop into the clinic less often. They may come by when in the area to say hello and to keep contact, but they know the treatment is over. We know the treatment is over for the time being. They will be back when another problem surfaces. With Samuel, we have heard through the grapevine, that he continues to attend classes in his own community and is receiving disability benefits. Is this a success? We think so. He is aware of the political nature of the benefits and he knows he is not crazy. He has established some age appropriate and not violent friendships. And, he knows the clinic is there if things get difficult again.

CONCLUSION

Clinical social work needs a paradigm shift. In order to solve the myriad of problems we face at the end of the Twentieth Century, on the individual to the national level (see Figure 1), we have to think differently; we have to think systemically. The more massive the breakdown of our social systems, institutions, and family structure, the greater the need to leap from the details of a smaller picture to the encompassing pattern. With both families and institutions, we need to find a pattern in the existing order that is working and then weave it into ever larger contexts. What currently works needs to be emphasized, otherwise, we will continue to feel swamped and paralyzed by focusing on all the parts that are not working.

What should be the role of social workers in the face of such widespread institutional breakdown? If social workers are to continue in a leadership role as champions of families we must advocate for a national family policy. We are the only major industrialized nation in the world that places the individual above family and community. We need to reassess our own thinking about health and illness, particularly with regard to the multi-cultural imperatives of the late Twentieth Century. Our models for training and treatment are largely predicated on a while, middle class value structure as it existed in a mono-cultural, stable world. None of these factors are valid as we reach the 1990s.

We need to use our clinical influence in our local communities and our political power on the state and national level to emphasize holistic and systemic thinking, not only as it applies to individuals and families, but as it applies to the entire relational system. We believe that it is imperative for clinicians of all disciplines, who have a firm grounding in systems thinking, to expand their horizons to include the larger domain and influence others who are still tying and untying their shoelaces.

BIBLIOGRAPHY

Alexander, P. (1985). A systems theory conceptualization of incest. *Family Process, 24*, 79-88.

Anderson, C. & Stewart, S. (1983). *Mastering resistance: A practical guide to family therapy*. New York: Guilford.

Carter, P. (1982). Rapport and integrity for Ericksonian practitioners. In J. Zeig, (Ed.), *Ericksonian approaches to hypnosis and psychotherapy*. New York: Brunner/Mazel.

Edelman, M.W. (1987). *Families in peril*. Cambridge: Harvard University Press.

Gleick, J. (1987). *Chaos*. New York: Viking Press.

Hartman, A., & Laird, J. (1983). *Family-centered social work practice*. New York: Free Press.

Imber-Black, E. (1988). *Families and larger systems: A family therapist's guide to family therapy*. New York: Guilford.

Kuhn, T. (1970). *The structure of scientific revolution*.

Lewis, K.G. (1989). The use of color-coded genograms in family therapy. *Journal of Marital and Family Therapy*, 15, 169-176.

McGoldrick, M., & Gerson, R. (1985). *Genograms in family assessment*. New York: W.W. Norton.

Moss-Kantor, R. (1989). *When giants learn to dance*. New York: Simon and Schuster.

Moynihan, D.P. (1986). *Family and nation*. New York: Harcourt Brace Jovanovich.

Parnell, M. & VanderKloot, J. (1989). Ghetto children: Children growing up in poverty. In L. Combrinck-Graham (Ed.), *Children in family contexts*. New York: Guilford Press.

Scheflin, A.E. (1981). *Levels of schizophrenia*. New York: Brunner/Mazel.

Sidel, R. (1986). *Women and children last*. New York: Viking Press.

Temas, R. (1990). The transfiguration of the western mind. *ReVision, 12* (3), 5.

Watzlawick, P., Weakland, J., & Fisch, R. (1974). *Change: Principles of problem formation and problem resolution*. New York: Norton.

Index

abusive behavior, 165-180
acculturation, 77
adoptee search organizations, 158, 160,161
adoption
  birth parents and, 155-158
  case illustrations, 151-155
  identity and, 158-161
  losses of, 151-158
  records of, 161
  reunification possibilities, 158
  social workers and, 149-162
  stories, 153-155
African-American communities
  AIDS in, 69-89
  changes in, 73-74
  crack epidemic in, 74-79
  distrust of outsiders, 71-72,73
  see also inner cities
African-American families
  extended families, 142,144-145
  foster care and, 135-146
  kinship bonds, 141-142
  strengths of, 81,141-142
AIDS (disease)
  in children, 75
  drug use and, 70,74-79
  ecosystemic approaches, 69-89
  gay community and, 69-70
  in minority communities, 69-89
  prevention programs, 72-73,79-83
  reasons for spread, 73-79
  silence surrounding, 70-72
American Family Therapy
    Association, 2
appointments, flexibility of, 194-195

assessment, clinical, 191-194
asylums, 122

babies, cocaine and, 86-89
battered women, 165-180
birth parents, 155-158
Black churches, 71,81
Black communities. *See* African-American communities
Black mothers. *See* mothers
Boston School of Social Work, 53
Brief Family Therapy Center, 111

case illustrations
  adoption, 151-155
  clinical assessment, 192-194
  eco-maps, 55,57
  homeless, 115-117
  social work training, 35-37
  urban poor treatment, 190-191, 195-201
Center for Disease Control, 71
changes
  in families, 43-45,49-50,61-64
  resistance to, 189-190
  rituals to mark, 64-66
  in social work students, 42-45, 48-50
chaos theory, 184-187,188,190
Child Welfare Association, 87,88
children
  AIDS and, 75
  development of shame, 167-170
  fighting among, 137-138
  in poverty, 75,77-78,137-138,187